Ms Blaelock's Book of Signature Wardrobe Planning

Also by Alexandria Blaelock

Ms Blaelock's Books
Stress Free Dinner Parties
Signature Wardrobe Planning
Holistic Personal Finance
Minimally Viable Housekeeping

Short Stories
Alma's Grace
Balancing the Book
Fate in Your Hands
Kiss of Death
Lady of the Looking Glass
Life in the Security Directorate
Long Weekend in the Snow
Love in the Security Directorate
Needy Bitch
Payton's Run
Phoenix Child
Shining Star
Ship in a Bottle
Simone Says Hands in the Air
The Guardian's Vigil
The Life and Death of Carmelita Basingstoke

Ms Blaelock's Book of Signature Wardrobe Planning

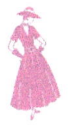

Alexandria Blaelock

BlueMere Books
MELBOURNE, AUSTRALIA

Copyright © 2015, 2020 by Alexandria Blaelock.

Originally published as Build Your Signature Wardrobe: How to look good and feel confident in four steps.

All rights reserved. No part of this publication may be reproduced, distributed or transmitted in any form or by any means, including photocopying, recording, or other electronic or mechanical methods, without the prior written permission of the publisher, except in the case of brief quotations embodied in critical reviews and certain other non-commercial uses permitted by copyright law.

For permission requests, contact enquiries@bluemerebooks.com.

Ordering Information:
Discounts are available on quantity purchases. For details, contact orders@bluemerebooks.com.

Signature Wardrobe Planning/Alexandria Blaelock.

hardback ISBN: 978-0-6481733-9-7
paperback ISBN: 978-0-9944415-8-4
digital ISBN: 978-0-9944415-9-1

Book Layout © 2015 BookDesignTemplates.com
Cover Image © RetroClipArt/Shutterstock.com

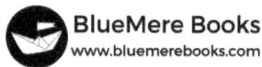

*In Loving Memory of Aunty M,
who told me I always look elegant.
(bless her).*

Style comes from knowing who you are and who you want to be in the world; it does not come from wanting to be somebody else, or wanting to be thinner, shorter, taller, prettier.

NINA GARCIA

Contents

Introduction	1
PART ONE: Historical Context	9
1900s	11
1910s	23
1920s	35
1930s	47
1940s	61
1950s	75
PART TWO: Develop Your Wardrobe Plan	87
Step 1: Set Your Budget	89
Step 2: Determine Your Appropriate	99
Step 3: Establish Your Style	111
Step 4: Decide Your Needs	127
Modern Day Worked Example	137
PART THREE: Build and Maintain Your Wardrobe	147
Record Keeping	149
How to Conduct a Wardrobe Review	159
How to Create a Capsule Wardrobe	169
What Good Fit Looks Like	177
What Good Quality Looks Like	189
Decoding Dress Codes	197
How to Choose a Hat	223
Let's Go Shopping!	209
Clothing Care	223
Maintaining Your Body	245
Glossary	253
Bibliography	265
Index	273
Author's Note	284
About the Author	285

Introduction

AS YOU SIT HERE TODAY, you are in many ways very fortunate. You could be invited to a gala event at a moment's notice, and if you are, you can go into any store and buy a new outfit: head to toe, inner to outer layers. Frock, shoes, bag, jewellery, makeup and an exotic new fragrance. You can visit a hairdresser for a fabulous do, get a mani-pedi and have your makeup done too. With very little thought and effort, you are dressed in an outfit worthy of an elegant soiree within hours.

You don't even need to consider whether you can afford it - just pull out your credit card and purchase whatever you need regardless of the price. Many of us would think looking perfect tonight is be more important than anything else.

Building a wardrobe that works over a longer term seems much more complicated than buying for a single event. At face value, buying a bunch of clothes seems quite straightforward. You can easily buy enough clothes to get you through a week without washing any of it, and they might even be fashionable.

However, it's more likely you've bought random stuff; not one garment matches any other, they aren't made from similar fibres, don't have common care instructions, and you can't comfortably wear them to any of the places you usually go.

So you are going to be paying them off for many months and probably won't wear them for even longer. You won't be "dressed", you'll just not be naked.

The advice given by the Woman's Institute of Domestic Arts and Sciences in 1925 is just as applicable today as then - don't cheat yourself or others by not dressing well. Be proud of yourself, dress to please yourself and enhance your confidence. "Make the time to learn what is appropriate, becoming and wholly lovely for you".

Just a few short decades ago, mass produced clothing wasn't readily obtainable, let alone affordable. It's hard to imagine, but up until the 1960s, people were generally reliant on clothes designed and manufactured in the country they were sold. Credit cards did not exist so shoppers were more careful, thought more deeply about what they needed, and shopped according to what they could afford.

I learnt to shop in the 80s, the early days of credit cards. Those days were so early we didn't understand the limit, thinking it was like a monthly allowance. My limit was $200, and that was about the amount I got paid each fortnight. Laughable now, but it seemed like a fortune to me. My employer supplied my uniform, so all I had to buy were what I like to call Princess Clothes - the ones I wore when I went out partying, looking for my Prince Charming.

Today, as always, the basic wardrobe planning problem is building this year's wardrobe on last year's clothes (not lack of money). I think this may be one of those universal truths so obvious you need someone to point it out. You need a process to ensure you buy clothes that work for the life you currently live, at a price you can afford.

While you'd probably LOVE to throw out all your clothes and start again, you can (and really should) start where you are. You wouldn't knock your house down to renovate your kitchen, you'd examine its current state, work out what is and isn't working, then plan and undertake the renovation work.

In just the same way, examining your clothes to understand what's working, what's not, and why you have nothing to wear gives you the information you need to make your plan. Then you can shop in the full and certain knowledge you'll require tremendous reserves of inner strength to stick with your plan.

This book comes in three parts.
1. Historical Context
2. Develop Your Wardrobe Plan
3. Build and Maintain Your Wardrobe

1: Historical Context

We start with an overview of the social and fashion conditions for each decade of the early twentieth century. While I have grouped the information into nice easy to absorb eras, fashion like most facets of life follows an evolutionary path and is not easily segmented.

I draw against statistical data relating to white working and middle class income and expenditure in the United States (US) and the United Kingdom (UK), simply because this information is easiest to find. So when I mention replacing a suit in three to four years, it's a figure based on what real people actually spent averaged out across the population. It's not that they were only *allowed* one suit every three years, it's just what they could afford to buy.

During the 59 years covered, there were changes in the statistical classification of people and purchases, as well as changes in the variety of goods available for purchase *and* the way people shopped not captured by the data. This accounts for some of the variation in whether jewellery, makeup, personal and clothing care costs are included in the clothing budget or not.

There are some inaccuracies due to different technological release dates between the US and the UK. This has resulted in some variations and inconsistencies within the information I've been able to access and provide for each decade.

As such, this overview is full of wild generalisations - across age, ethnicity, class, urban/rural and country. But as this part isn't intended to be a dryly accurate academic account of what your life might have been like during this time, I think that's fine. This part forms an introduction to the ways the prevailing economic conditions and standards of living at the time would impact your purchasing plan. Naturally some found it easier while others (non-whites in particular) were in a much more challenging position.

I provide this information to show you the way you dress is influenced more deeply by the larger world around you than you suspect. I hope this makes it easier to consider the place of appropriateness and style in your own wardrobe.

2: Develop Your Wardrobe Plan

Using fashion and shopping advice from 1900 - 1959 (the same time frame as the statistics) I'll guide you through a four-step process that gives you the information and confidence you need to make a plan and stick with it. I'll help you:

1. decide how much you can spend. You'll be brave enough to face the unpleasant truth you can't afford *all*

the nice things you want, and confident enough to make the hard decisions you must.
2. determine what clothes are appropriate for you right now in the life you currently lead, regardless of your age, size, location and occupation(s). Not the imaginary one where you're 20lb (9kg) lighter, or the one where you're a Princess with a house full of servants doing your bidding. But something comfortable for you no matter where you live or what you do.
3. work out what your style is, and how you can present your authentic self to the world in a deep and truly unique way. You will look good and feel confident while still fitting in with the expectations of others.
4. decide what clothes and accessories are necessary for you, and how many of them you require. You will understand how to put together the most practical, functional and cost effective wardrobe possible.

3: Build and Maintain Your Wardrobe

I will help you navigate the mysteries of putting your wardrobe plan into action. You will learn:

- what sorts of records to keep and why
- how to review your wardrobe
- what the different kinds of capsule wardrobes are, and which one is best for you
- clothes don't fit when you try them because there is something wrong with them (not you!), and what you can do about it
- what the characteristics of quality are and how you can prioritise them
- what clothes to wear for a variety of dress code occasions; historic and contemporary

- how to shop efficiently and effectively
- how to take care of your clothes so you can maximise their lifespans

There's some repetition between the Develop Your Wardrobe Plan and Build and Maintain You Wardrobe parts, but only so you have the relevant information to hand and don't need to keep flicking backwards and forwards to find it.

In this book, I use the term wardrobe to refer to your clothes, and closet for the places you put them. I've also put a glossary at the end, so if you come across a word or abbreviation you don't understand (or forget) you can look it up.

The matrix shown on the next page provides examples of the different kinds of clothes I refer to through this book.

Signature Wardrobe Planning

Table 1: Historical Clothing Styles

	Daywear high necklines and long sleeves plain wool and cotton	**Eveningwear** low necklines and short sleeves luxurious and embellished fabrics
House Clothes (wear in private)	work (chores)	leisurewear (relaxing)
Street Clothes (wear in public)	career socialising church galleries, museums sportswear	dinner parties concerts, theatre gala functions

Are you ready? Then turn the page and let's get started!

PART ONE:
Historical Context

THIS PART GIVES AN IDEA of the constraints people worked within when they were planning their wardrobes. If you want to get straight to business, skip this section and go to Part Two (Develop Your Wardrobe Plan).

CHAPTER 1

1900s

THE NEW CENTURY SEEMED FULL of promise, with new technologies offering better ways of doing things and never-ending advances in science.

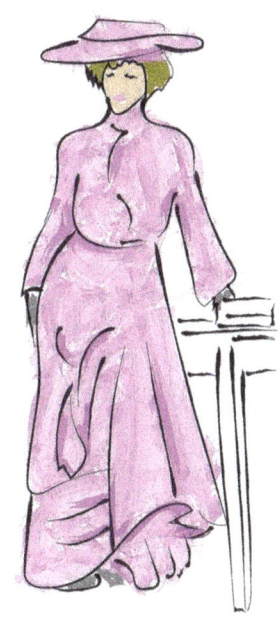

ON THE WORLD STAGE

Politics

At the turn of the twentieth century, Queen Victoria died and the British throne passed to her son Edward (VII). He and his pals enjoyed European fashions and art which led to a distinctive design style generally referred to as Edwardian. Australia gained self-rule; Cuba, Norway and Bulgaria gained independence, and the Irish demanded home rule.

War

The first decade of the twentieth century wasn't peaceful, with the Boer War (resulting in British annexation of the free republics), the Philippine-American War (of Independence) and the Russo-Japanese War for control of Manchuria and Korea. Plus the Russian Revolution and the Herero War genocide.

Disaster

The planet was rocked by hurricanes in Galveston, typhoons in Hong Kong, earthquakes in Guatemala, San Francisco, Jamaica, and Italy as well as volcanic eruptions in Martinique and Italy. There were disastrous fires in Ottawa, the Hoboken docks, Jacksonville, the Paris Metro, the Iroquois Theatre Chicago, Baltimore and the steamboat General Slocum. Ocean liners SS Norge and SS Valencia sank, and there was an explosion at the Rolling Mill Mine.

Science and Technology

Scientific and technological advancements included Einstein's theory of *special* relativity, and the development of the seismograph, air conditioner, Geiger counter, alkaline battery, electric typewriter, dictation machine, radio receiver and broadcaster. Additionally, the neon lamp, lie detector, continuous tractor tracks, Photostat machine, Bakelite, the first Zeppelin and aeroplane flights, and the tuberculosis vaccination.

Domestic Developments

On the domestic front, petrol and diesel cars entered mass production. Phonographs and gramophones became popular home entertainments. You could buy low-cost brownie cameras, clocks that made tea, and pianola devices that played recordings made by pianists.

The Arts

"Popular" music was just beginning its separation from "Classical" with recordings of singers generally supported by orchestras. Popular songs included *Take Me Out to the Ballgame*, *Pomp and Circumstance* and *Anchors Aweigh*. In the literary world, publications included *The Wizard of Oz*, *The Call of the Wild*, *Anne of Green Gables*, and *The Secret Agent*. With the invention of cinema came *The Great Train Robbery* and the first feature film *The Story of the Kelly Gang*. Art movements included Post-Impressionism (Van Gogh), Symbolism (Gauguin) and Art Nouveau (Klimt).

SOCIAL AND TECHNOLOGICAL DEVELOPMENTS IN FASHION

Social Expectations

Upper class women embraced leisure activities which led to the development of less restrictive clothing, though corsets and long skirts were still worn every day. Bicycles had been available since the late 1880s, and women were using them to get around. Bloomer dresses (a very loose pant that looked like a skirt when standing) were losing popularity, but looser corsets and shorter skirts remained.

Changes in transport technologies led to changes in dress; cars in the 1900s were open and required protection for clothing, and as more women started driving, their skirts became a little shorter. In 1904, drivers were advised to wear leather for warmth and wind protection, punched for summer to promote air circulation and evaporation of perspiration. Headwear was essential, and women were advised to wear veils to secure their hats and protect their faces from dust. Duster coats were developed for rain protection.

Aeroplanes were also open to the elements, making goggles essential. Female fliers needed to have their skirts tied to their legs and many women aviators wore men's leather jackets, helmets, breeches and boots instead.

In the early 1900s, swimwear for women was pantaloons with a dress, an outfit that effectively prevented swimming even had it been socially acceptable. In 1905 Annette Kellerman (aged 18), a well-known Australian swimmer and diver was invited to perform in London for the Royal Family. She was accustomed to competing in a man's one piece tank suit that exposed her thighs, but as this was forbidden by the venue she sewed black stockings onto her suit for the performance. She was arrested for indecency in Boston in 1907 for swimming in her man's suit, but was permitted by the judge to wear it while swimming for health benefits, providing she wore a robe when not in the water. This outfit became the "Annette Kellermanns" women's swimsuit; a man's suit with the addition of a fitted skirt worn over the top for modesty.

The first permanent hair wave was developed around 1906, it was a process involving chemicals *and* electrically produced heat and took about 10 hours in the beauty salon.

Signature Wardrobe Planning

Fabric Developments

Favoured fabrics were crepe de chine, chiffon, mousseline and tulle in pink, blue and mauve pastels. Some satin dresses were embroidered or painted in tiny floral patterns.

The first manufactured fibre of the twentieth century was viscose. It was marketed as artificial silk because it drapes, stretches and shrinks like silk (renamed rayon in 1924) and is still used as a silk substitute today.

It's manufactured from very short cotton fibres or wood chips, dissolved, mixed with chemicals and the resulting solution filtered and forced into a sulphuric acid bath that triggers the production of long cellulose fibres. It comes in several variants; viscose rayon, rayon or viscose. Cuprammonium rayon is another form of rayon; as its manufacture is an environmentally harmful process it is now difficult to obtain.

The second fibre is a relative of rayon; it's also made from cotton or wood, but uses a different chemical process to result in cellulose acetate. Acetate looks shiny and is often found in formal and bridal gowns and decorative fabrics. The fibre was called acetate silk until 1924, rayon until 1953 and is now known as acetate.

Sewing Machines

The sewing machine as we know it today was in general use in the home by 1900. Most working class women were sewing their family's clothes by hand in the nineteenth century. An experienced sewer could make an average shirt with 20,620 stitches in 10 - 14 hours at the rate of 35 stitches per minute. Using a machine that sewed 3,000 stitches a minute on average reduced the task to one hour.

At this time, you could order a drop head treadle machine for $10 from a catalogue, or a Singer sewing machine from a travelling salesman for $40 - $75.

Manufacturing

While menswear was almost exclusively ready-to-wear, most middle class women's clothing was still made-to-measure. The orders were generally taken by a catalogue, salon, or at one of the new-fangled department stores and made up in a sweat-shop or as piecework by a dressmaker working from home.

The working conditions some seamstresses worked in were so bad that trade boards were set up in the UK to regulate them. Should you be wealthy enough to travel to Paris, the same circumstances would apply, though your day dresses may have been made by a dressmaker who came to the house to measure you up.

Working class women generally made their own clothes; with sewing machines if they could afford them.

MEANWHILE AT HOME

If you were alive in the early twentieth century, you would not have had mains running water, gas or electricity.

Housing

Rental shortages meant tenants couldn't be too fussy - few homes had toilets, even less running water. Indoor toilets and kitchens with sinks were the minimum standards for the middle class, but the height of luxury for working class - only 20% of New York families had a bathroom though 31% had a toilet in their apartment.

Water Supply

You may have had a rainwater tank connected to a tap inside the house, but most likely would have had to take eight or ten trips each day to a dam, creek or spring, well or town pump to fill the tank up.

Doing the Laundry

Doing the laundry would have been gruelling hard work, and one load of washing (washed, boiled and rinsed) would use about 50 gallons (190L) of water.

To start, you and your family would change clothes on Sunday - you would sort by colour, fabric and level of soil before soaking your fine (delicate) whites overnight in warm water with a little soap grated or scraped from the bar before any stains could set.

Then on Monday you got up early and got to work.

1. Lay out all your tubs - a second washing tub, one for boiling, one for rinsing with plain water, one for bluing rinse, and one for starch.

2. Put some water on to heat up, and grate some soap while you wait. You might have had a wood or coal stove, but many working class families still relied on open fires.

3. Drain your fine whites.

4. Pour hot suds over them before rubbing them on your washboard.

5. Wring them out and apply soap directly to stubborn stains.

6. Cover them with fresh water and bring to the boil. While you are waiting, put your coarse whites to soak in the water leftover from the fine whites if it doesn't look too dirty.

7. Stir your fine whites while they are boiling so they don't go yellow.

8. When your clothes are done, remove, rub any remaining stains with soap.

9. Rinse in plain water and wring out.

10. Rinse the whites in a bluing agent to make them look whiter and wring again.

11. Dip in starch for stiffness or body (especially collars), and wring out.

12. Carry washing outside to hang on the line to dry.

13. When dry, take down and fold ready for ironing.

14. Replenish the water heating on the stove and exchange any water too dirty to reuse.

15. If necessary pop back to the well for more fresh water.

16. Then repeat the above with your coarse whites.

17. And your colours.

18. Finish with your woollen underwear.

And in between, tend your livestock and vegetable garden, mind the kids and prepare food.

Tuesday is your day for ironing.

1. Put a clean sheet of iron on the fire to heat.

2. Set at least two, but perhaps three to six irons of varying weights on the iron to heat.

3. Dampen your dry clothes, roll them in a cloth and leave them until the irons are hot enough.

Signature Wardrobe Planning

4. Cover your table, shirt, and skirt ironing boards with a woollen ironing cloth so they are ready when you need them.

5. When hot, rub your iron with beeswax to prevent sticking, wipe clean and test on paper or rags to make sure it's not too hot.

6. Iron like mad while it's still hot before putting it back on the sheet to reheat.

7. Wax, clean and test the second one.

8. Swap for heavier irons when you need more weight for thicker fabric and lighter irons for thinner.

9. Continue ironing every single garment you have washed because all your clothes are cotton or wool (that's just how they come) and they all need ironing. And because you are a proud woman and don't want anyone thinking you aren't taking proper care of your family.

Many urban poor families had no choice but to send out their laundry because they did not have space or the equipment to wash their own clothes, particularly when it came to men's shirts and collars.

INCOME AND CLOTHING EXPENDITURE

Income

At this time husbands, wives and children all worked for pay. Some households also took in boarders or lodgers, and some had income from other sources including home grown produce. The average annual wage in 1905 was:

- Working Class: $497
- Middle Class: $720

Clothing Expenditure

The first survey of retail prices was published in 1903, and this showed households spent 14% of their income on clothing. However, this data group also includes carpets, horse blankets, leather hides and wool fleeces so it's likely the actual clothing spend was less. As prices increased by 12% over the course of the decade, the proportional cost of income may have increased. The family spend was split 32% on the husband, 27% for the wife and 41% towards children's clothing.

Womenswear

Key Looks

The decade started with stiff S shape corsets and high collars though this still premitted different outfits for different kinds of activities. Within this silhouette were two basic stereotypes:

- John Singer Sargent's idealised portraits of upper class women with their open necks, tiny waists and up-dos.

- Charles Dana Gibson's pen and ink sketches of ordinary young women with pigeon bosoms, nipped in waists and hobble skirts.

The decade became a debate about what a beautiful woman was; the painted ideal or the real woman captured in a moment of time by a photograph. It was the start of the realisation that beauty was more elusive than having the right clothes and jewels, it was a different kind of quality.

Middle class women new to the workforce in respectable roles as governesses and typists wore "professional" tailored dresses whereas non-working women wore skirts with floppy lacy blouses.

Key Figures

While some actors and dancers were becoming more socially acceptable, without radio, television or the internet, they had little influence. Newspapers were available, and then as now scandal sheets were popular, but entertainers were not "celebrities" and not generally thought newsworthy. In any case, ordinary people had little money for discretionary purposes and tended to dress for practicality.

Key Designers

Conservative wealthy women had their clothes made-to-measure at the House of Worth (the first couturier to offer bespoke clothing in Paris) famous for beautiful and finely detailed design and execution. More adventurous women went to Callot Soeurs for traditional silhouettes enhanced with exotic Eastern influences like harem pants and kimono sleeves in metallic fabrics encrusted with jewels.

Later in the decade, designers started relaxing the corset's S shape. Jeanne Paquin designed more functional, yet beautifully delicate dresses with empire lines, hidden pleats and fur or lace trimmings.

Paul Poiret developed a more comfortable and beautiful free-flowing silhouette created by draping rather than tailoring. He is best known for the kimono coat, hobble skirts, harem pants and the straight silhouette. He was among the first designers to add a perfume line and set up their own fabric house to develop fabrics and decorative arts in support of their clothing lines. Some of these employed designers and/or artists who were inspired by events such as the discovery of Tutankhamen's tomb or Indonesian batik patterns.

Stores like Liberty of London commissioned fabrics and designs to challenge the French dominance.

CHAPTER 2

1910s

THE 1910S WERE A DECADE of tumultuous changes, the passing of one way of life and the beginning of the modern era.

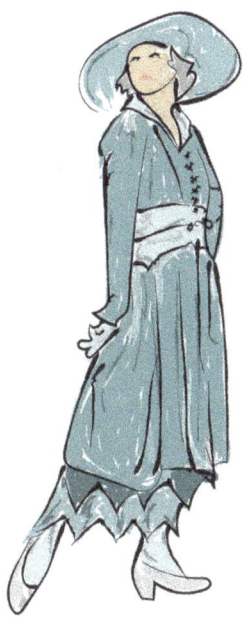

ON THE WORLD STAGE

Politics

The German monarchy was abolished in favour of the elected government of the Weimar Republic, George V succeeded Edward VII to the British throne, and the war-torn European and Asian states began reorganising themselves. In the US, the Temperance movement had a big win with the introduction of Prohibition in 1919.

War

The decade's main conflict was, of course, the First World War (the Great War) spanning 1914 - 19, but the Wadai War, First Balkan Wars and War of Latvian independence also took place at this time. Additionally, the Russian, Xinhai and Mexican Revolutions, and the British slaughter of peaceful protesters in the Jallianwala Bagh.

Disaster

Two years of Spanish Flu killed millions, the Netherlands was flooded by a North Sea storm, the Japanese volcano Sakurajima erupted, and there were shark attacks on the Jersey Shore. The Ocean liners RMS Titanic and RMS Lusitania sank.

Science and Technology

Scientific and technological developments included Einstein's theory of *general* relativity, the invention of stainless steel, the zipper and the Tank.

Domestic Developments

Domestically, the invention of the pop-up toaster and crossword, plus the general availability and use of radio receivers.

The Arts

This was the era of the first Jazz record. Books included *Sons and Lovers*, *Tarzan of the Apes*, *Pygmalion*, *Death in Venice* and *Wild Fire*. Movies included *Oliver Twist*, *The Musketeers of Pig Alley*, and the first appearances of Charlie Chaplin's little tramp. Artistic movements included Cubism (Picasso), Expressionism (Munch) and Futurism (Marinetti).

In Other News

Hiram Bingham rediscovered Machu Picchu, and the Panama Canal was completed.

SOCIAL AND TECHNOLOGICAL DEVELOPMENTS IN FASHION

Social Expectations

Clothing indicated both class and gender. It was still formal but men were choosing soft over stiff collars and women's skirts were getting shorter. Status items such as watches and jewellery were becoming important for older middle class children. Generally husbands spent more on quality and variety while wives bought higher status. Working class families needed replacements while the middle class sought improvements.

Clothing styles were significantly affected by fabric rationing and labour shortages during the First World War, as well as the need for clothing that provided greater freedom of movement. Jersey (a stretchy knitted fabric previously restricted to underwear and workwear) became a functional part of many wardrobes, and the first brassiere was invented.

After women's swimming events were added to the 1912 Olympics, it was increasingly accepted as a healthy pursuit for women, however aside from competition, women's swimsuits were closer to the 1900 pantaloons than the Kellermans.

When enclosed cars became more common, women gave up parasols and large hats and started wearing wristwatches.

Fabric Developments

Natural fibres were still almost the only ones available and so the majority of fabrics consisted of woven cotton, linen, silk and wool though rayon was becoming popular, as were jersey knits. Rayon was coming into full production in household goods as well as hosiery and clothing.

Sewing Machines

In 1915, Singer patented a new machine head and subsequently launched the 101, a gear driven, top bobbin rotary machine built for electrical operation. It had a built-in motor and light, and completely encased lower mechanism. It was quiet with almost no vibration, but over time slowed down and couldn't be repaired adequately. While the general focus of this decade was reducing the machine weight, generally by releasing smaller versions, Singer introduced the first vertical system sewing machine (the 115) with a vertical semi-oscillating shuttle system in 1917.

Manufacturing

Men's ready-to-wear expanded from the department store to become more widely available at gentleman's outfitters. Traditionally tailors had made an entire garment, but technological advances in cutting and sewing made it possible to factory manufacture clothing.

New York's Triangle Shirtwaist factory combined the most modern equipment with the most antiquated sweatshop practices. In 1911, the factory caught fire and 146 people, mainly women and migrant workers, died after being locked in the building. Following the incident, the industry became divisive with strikes and factory floor unionisation across the New York and Chicago garment districts.

The resulting inquiry led to landmark changes in safety and sanitary conditions, collective bargaining, and limitations on women and children's working hours. The men who owned the factory were acquitted of manslaughter by an all-male jury.

MEANWHILE AT HOME

Men faced long working days, and their wives gruelling household chores with a trip to the movies almost the only escape.

Housing

Home ownership was increasing across all classes though the middle class was more likely to live in a larger house with a yard than an apartment.

Regardless of layout or what the landlord claimed, the general practice across class was to use two rooms for communal living (kitchen, dining and living), one for the parents to sleep in and whatever was left for the children. When older children were old enough to receive guests, one of the sleeping rooms would have been converted to a reception room (dining or parlour) and the living room adapted for sleeping as well.

Water Supply

Most homes had at least cold running water and access to a toilet. The middle class had an inside toilet and a bathroom, but the working class would have shared their earth closet and not had water in the bathroom. While plumbing manufacture and installation started as specialist fields, mass production improvements over the first three decades of the twentieth century moved plumbing accessibility further down the income scale and most people had running water by the mid-thirties.

Doing the Laundry

The needs of the commercial laundry industry led to the development of electric machines that could agitate clothes in warm soapy water, contained within two concentric cylinders (which remains the basis of most modern machines). They required manual intervention to start, stop, add soap, add and remove water, and feed into the attached wringer.

Domestic washing machines started to become available, but for poorer households these remained human-powered crank handled machines that mimicked the use of a washboard, with a crank-handled wringer.

You still had to carry the water and manually soak, boil, rinse, blue and starch the clothes, but these two machines significantly reduced the time and effort required to do the laundry. Particularly in combination with newly available pre-prepared washing soap; Lux flakes in 1906 and Rinso granulated in 1918.

Around 60% of working class families sent some laundry out, and about 70% of middle class families did too, but the bulk was still washed at home - electric machines reduced labour and dependence on outside help. But the old methods still worked better on natural fibres.

Gas Supply

Mass production also allowed Sears to make wood or coal fired stoves and furnaces for household heating and hot water available around 1908. These fuels were quite labour intensive with carrying, stacking, tending fires and cleaning stoves. Fuel consumption increased by class; the wealthier the family, the more likely to use an easier source of fuel.

Coal provided 70% of the energy consumed, but it came in various forms. Bituminous coal was the dirtiest and cheapest (22 - 24% of budget) therefore, the most consumed providing 40 - 44% of British Thermal Units (BTU). Anthracite coal provided 28% of BTU for 21% of the household budget.

Gas was mainly used for lighting (not cooking or heating). It provided 20% of BTU for 25% of budget. Facing competition from kerosene and electricity, gas lighting companies aligned with manufacturers of gas stoves, water heaters, fridges, coolers and dishwashers. A major advertising campaign over 1912 - 13 had assured gas future by 1918.

Electricity Supply

Electricity was enormously expensive and mainly used for lighting. Middle class households spent on average 14% more on fuel and used 14% more BTU (bought more energy that was cleaner and easier to use). They used more of all forms of energy than the working class. There were, of course, city and regional variations affecting fuel needs due to changes in climate, housing design and size, and sanitation needs.

Both alternating current (AC) and direct current (DC) was available, with products for either and both available into the 1930s. In 1912, 16% of American homes had electricity connected though it was really only affordable by those who could also afford servants. And with a shortage of those, by 1917 the middle class were buying electrical "servants" to sew, wash and iron their clothes. Other popular appliances included fans, dishwashers and carpet sweepers.

As electricity spread, its price fell, but while people bought more appliances and installed more lights, electric cooking was still rare. By 1920, half of non-farm dwellings had electricity though poorer families used less of it.

INCOME AND CLOTHING EXPENDITURE

Income

In 1918, employed wives were uncommon, but while working class wives were the most likely to work, they only earned about a third of their husband's wages. Counterintuitively, working class children were least likely to work for pay but when they did, they made about 20% of their father's wage. Around 40% - 45% of families had additional income from produce and/or livestock. Some had income from investments, and as you would expect this was more likely in the middle classes. Government income support did not exist. The average annual household income (from all sources) in 1918 was:

- Working Class: $1,037
- Middle Class: $1,344
- Upper Class: $2,272

Clothing Expenditure

Clothing prices escalated as demand increased while global production of raw materials and the availability of finished items decreased due to the First World War. Other constraints included difficulty shipping and the cessation of trade relationships with some countries during hostilities.

Signature Wardrobe Planning

In 1917, the US Government instituted a regulatory scheme to protect the interests of the government and civilians by ensuring production and controlling prices. In practice, the priority placed on government war matériels led to civilian shortages and high prices.

During this decade, there was an ideological battle between modesty and frugality (championed by Ellen Richards, leading American home economist and Massachusetts Institute of Technology sanitary chemistry instructor), and the comfortable enjoyment of the fruits of your labour (Martha Bruère, one time Good Housekeeping editor and writer of financial advice articles).

As shown over the page, the recommended clothing allocation spanned 8 - 20% depending on income and family size.

Table 2: Comparison of Annual Household Clothing Budgets Richards (1910) and Bruère (1912)

	Income	Budget
Richards	$800 - $2,000	15%
	$2,000 - $4,000	20%
Bruère	Allison $1,800 (young couple)	12.5%
	Wells $2,400 (3 adult children)	8%
	Parnell $4,000 (4 young children)	11.25%

As their public roles were smaller, almost all additional and unexpected costs were deducted from the wife's clothing allowance, first her street clothes and then replacement house clothes. Generally the expenditure for husbands and working children were the same, and about 20% less for wives. As income increased, the disparity between the parents reduced.

Cleaning, repairs and shoes accounted for about 12% of the budget, with a larger proportion for the husband, and greater usage and expenditure by the middle class.

Womenswear

Key Looks

"Empire" gowns with slim hips were a popular choice, and when worn with large hats had the effect of slimming the hips further. They came in vivid colours and soft draping. As the decade progressed, skirts passed through a hobble phase (and some women wore restraints to prevent them from taking large steps and tearing their dresses) and then tapered further giving the silhouette of a triangle balanced on its point.

The decade also saw the arrival of the V neck, at the time considered both indecent *and* a health risk, but increasingly popular nonetheless. The two layered skirt (ankle length underskirt with knee length overskirt) was also introduced.

Once war broke out, clothing became less extravagant with simpler lines that used less fabric.

Key Figures

The *Ballet Russes* launched in 1909 and spent most of the decade touring Europe. The company caused a sensation with its ground breaking dance style and collaborations with young composers and artists. Their bright and exotically decorated folk and modern art based costumes captured the imagination.

More accessible dancers like Isadora Duncan and Martha Graham with their lithe muscular bodies provided inspiration for loose unstructured clothing and diaphanous gowns that made women's bodies more visible as the decade progressed.

Movies were becoming a common leisure activity, and as more people saw more movies, actresses became more influential style icons. However, money was tight so most women wore old clothes and merely dreamt of replacing them with something like they saw on the big screen. Theda Bara became the first sex symbol with her movie femme fatale persona, in contrast to America's Sweetheart Mary Pickford, and dancer Irene Castle who made close contact dancing respectable.

Key Designers

Madeleine Vionnet took inspiration from Ancient Greek and Roman statuary, and Mariano Fortuny pioneered silk painting and pleating. Naturally, these techniques were so carefully guarded that some, like Fortuny's signature dyed and pleated Delphos gowns have been lost.

Lucile (Lady Lucy Duff-Gordon) brought the delicacy of lingerie to street clothes, as well as unstructured underwear and tea dresses.

Jeanne Lanvin set rich colours, complex trim and ornamentation such as embroidery and beading in simple silhouettes. Many of her styles were inspired by historical figures and used petticoats and panniers.

The personality of the designer was becoming an important component of attracting buyers and making sales.

CHAPTER 3

1920s

THE ROARING 1920S FUELLED THE promise of a consumer society liberated by the automobile. Women achieved economic, social and political liberation, and this was reflected by the simple flat lines of their modern wardrobes.

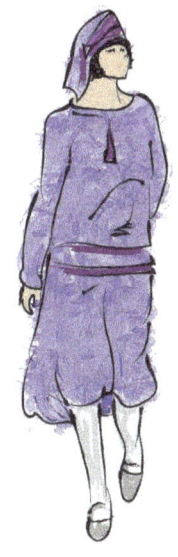

ON THE WORLD STAGE

Politics

In the 1920s, women in the UK and the US gained the right to vote. In the US, immigration restrictions were implemented, Ku Klux Klan membership reached its peak, and a Tennessee school teacher was fined $100 for illegally teaching evolution. The Irish Free State and Egypt gained independence.

In Europe, fascism rose in opposition to communism, with Mussolini becoming the Italian Prime Minister in 1922. Hyperinflation in the Weimar Republic led to the French occupation of its main industrial region to preserve the (outgoing) flow of war reparations, which in turn triggered the formation of the National Socialist German Workers' (Nazi) Party.

War

The Twenties are generally thought of as a decade of peace and prosperity, but during this time the Turkish War of Independence, the Polish-Soviet War, the Irish Civil War and Castellammarese Wars all took place.

Disaster

The stock market crashed on October 29, 1929.

Science and Technology

Developments included the cathode ray tube, the electrical phonograph recording process, the first liquid-fuelled rocket flight, jukeboxes and the negative feedback amplifier.

Domestic Developments

Domestically, inventions included the electric razor, television followed by the colour television were invented. Clarence

Birdseye developed his frozen food process. Popular pastimes include dancing, mah-jong, crosswords and pole-sitting (exactly what it sounds like - sitting on a pole. As a test of endurance. Of all things...).

The Arts

Jazz was still popular, particularly composer George Gershwin (my favourite), played by commercial radio stations in the US and the BBC in the UK.

Books included *The Great Gatsby*, *Winnie-the-Pooh*, *A Farewell to Arms*, *Lady Chatterley's Lover*, *Ulysses*, and *All Quiet on the Western Front*.

Sound movies became available; *Don Juan* (with a record), part talking *The Jazz Singer*, all talking *Lights of New York*, colour talkie *On with the Show*, and the last silent film *Modern Times*.

Artistic movements include Surrealism (Dali), Abstract (Kandinsky), Modernism (Chagall), Fauvism (Matisse), and Neoplasticism (Mondrian).

In Other News

Manhattan's Museum of Modern Art opened to the public and Howard Carter uncovered Tutankhamun's tomb. Charles Lindbergh took the first solo flight across the Atlantic.

SOCIAL AND TECHNOLOGICAL DEVELOPMENTS IN FASHION

Social Expectations

After the First World War, social expectations relaxed as women needed to be able to travel independently for work.

While the working class bought ready-to-wear, the middle classes enjoyed made-to-measure copies of Paris fashion. The upper class continued to purchase haute couture for their eveningwear and hired a dressmaker for their daywear though couturiers were starting to offer complete wardrobes of day and evening clothes.

During this time, France was still the centre of fashion, and even though the London and New York fashion industries were flourishing, they drew against Paris fashions as a matter of course. Couturiers sold "official models" for duplication by top tier stores such as Harrods and Macys, as well as "bonded models" as a source for cheaper copies or paper patterns to manufacturers and ready-to-wear retailers. Store owners and manufacturers visited France seeking inspiration, and the upper class made seasonal buying trips.

At this time, sportswear found a permanent place in the wardrobe. This was originally a term for clothing worn during sporting activities but was broadening to include watching sport and is now commonly used to describe a uniquely American style of casual dress. These clothes were originally designed for outdoor pursuits such as golf, horse riding, skiing, and so on, that were previously undertaken in the usual restrictive corseted daywear.

They were comfortable clothes, generally knitted with simple masculine tailored lines and popularised by the relaxed clothes worn by actresses Katherine Hepburn and Marlene Dietrich - particularly pants. The range also included clothing such as long coats, gloves and hats.

With the introduction of enclosed cars and aircraft cabins, along with comfortable seating in 1919, passenger travel became more commonplace in the 1920s and fashionable sportswear became the standard dress code for travel.

In 1926, Gertrude Ederle became the first woman to swim the English Channel in a suit similar to the Kellermanns, making functional swimsuits socially acceptable. As women swimming in public became more usual, public pools became family spaces, and women "Bathing Belles".

Inspired by the high contrast seen on movie screens, many women started wearing visible makeup. Cosmetics were only just openly sold and lipstick, rouge, mascara and nail polish became common. The first eyelash curler was invented in 1923.

Cosmetic and reconstructive surgery has its roots in the 1920s treatment of post-war facial wounds, and Fanny Brice famously became the first celebrity to have a nose job in 1923.

With shortening hems (knee length in 1925) and sleeves, it became customary for women to remove visible body hair from legs and armpits. Shorter dresses made feet a focal point and women chose coloured shoes with high heels, T-bars, crossed over straps or embellishments such as cut outs, embroideries and beads in preference to practical walking boots.

Fabric Developments

Manufactured fibre fabrics were not yet common, and the majority of clothes were still made from cotton, linen, wool and silk in blends and different finishes.

Rayon had been on sale since 1911 and experienced rapid growth throughout the 1920s due to its low-cost luxury look, and its ability to meet the fashion for soft lines, draping and vivid colours. Silk stockings became more affordable after the war and replaced cotton as the standard for everyday wear.

Sewing Machines

The US Office of Home Economics conducted studies examining the amount of physical labour required to complete housework. They determined that using an electric machine and hand sewing required the same amount of energy per hour, but that an electric machine could complete 16 times more work. The treadle machine used six times more energy than hand sewing but resulted in 14 times more work.

The fashion for simple sack dresses meant more women could make their own clothes at home. Advertising also encouraged them to think that home sewing was an important act of domestic economy and the pursuit of fashion was morally acceptable. In general, most women made their own clothes supplemented by difficult to produce ready-to-wear items such as stockings, jewellery and other accessories.

Sewing machines were available as cabinet style manual machines and as standalone appliances in boxes, and could be wired for AC or DC current. The drive for lighter, smaller and quieter machines continued.

Manufacturing

Simple lines also meant that the burgeoning ready-to-wear clothing industry could increase production to meet the needs of a growing market. It was cheap and readily available through mail order and chain stores, though without standard sizing the perfect fit remained the domain of haute couture.

Two kinds of plastics became available in the 20s; thermoplastic (softens with heat) and thermoset (does not). Bakelite (patented in 1909) a thermoset material, became very fashionable in jewellery during the 1920s and 30s Art Deco period. Plastics were more widely used in buttons and belts as well as footwear and hair accessories as the decade progressed.

Meanwhile at Home

High levels of post-war consumer demand improved the conditions of working class families, but they still lived in dark cramped apartments, mended clothing, and walked a lot, with Church their primary social activity. Despite this, many still had to make some hard choices about household expenditure.

Housing

Home ownership was not common, and many people shared houses with other families. While houses consisting of two rooms were still common, the expectation of city dwellers was a minimum of four rooms with bath and running water for a family of five. Heated apartments were available, but unheated was the most common. Less urban residences might have a private earth closet in the yard, but some would have been shared between several houses.

Single people working in the city commonly took a room at something like the Young Men's or Women's Christian Associations. In larger cities they ate in restaurants rather than at their boarding houses, though young women may have prepared some or all of their food in their rooms.

Families living in homes with yards still grew fruit and vegetables and kept chickens and cows where possible for food and supplementary income.

Water Supply

While plumbed water was becoming more common in larger cities (to a sink in the kitchen), many families still relied on local or town wells. City apartments were available with a range of plumbing depending on what you could afford. Not all buildings had water connected, and those that did were not always plumbed through to all the apartments; the lowest rent had none, mid-range just cold while the highest rents had hot.

Doing the Laundry

In areas where electricity and plumbing were available, washing machines were very popular - in 1921 70% of washing machines were electric, increasing to 84% by 1929. Single men generally paid their boarding houses around $1 a week for laundry and clothing repairs, and single women $1.25.

Most wives washed their clothes at home, though when she was ill, old, or lacked access to utilities, she would get help in (a cleaning or washing lady cost around $3 per day) or send laundry out.

Gas Supply

Houses without electricity and gas relied on oil or kerosene for lighting. Wood and coal were still standard for heating and cooking. Domestic users were a very small market for gas, comprising wealthy people who could afford the high cost of plumbing and fuel.

Electricity Supply

By late 1929 85% of non-farm households had electricity. Only 10% of farms had electricity, but 25% of those had electric washing machines. The electric iron was the most popular appliance during the 1920s, with the first adjustable automatic thermostat model on sale in 1927. Some houses had electricity connected, but not water.

Telephone

Telephones were not common; on call and supervisory staff may have had company phones installed in their homes.

INCOME AND CLOTHING EXPENDITURE

Income

During the war, employment opportunities had expanded for both working and middle class women, in some cases she became the family breadwinner. These women with greater means could now afford to consider fashion as well as practicality and cost in their clothing choices.

Despite increasing employment in stores and offices, the mainstay of women's work was domestic or farm service. As city girls moved into retail and clerical work, the gap in domestic service was filled by country girls moving to the city. Anecdotal evidence suggests that domestic service was seen as more respectable and secure, with potential for promotion or improvement. The annual average wage for 1925 was:

- Working Class: $1,174
- Middle Class: $1,705

Clothing Expenditure

Around this time, women started to buy or make more "good" dresses, for some lucky women as many as four new dresses each season, giving them the opportunity to dress according to their mood. Of course, they still needed to shop for practicality and not sentimentality.

In 1920, shoppers were advised to practice economy in clothes shopping by considering a garment's practicality for promoting health, its durability, quality, and that its design lines were plain enough to allow use over several seasons. The recommended allocation for clothing spanned 10.8% - 20.23% of income depending on income and family size.

You were expected to undertake a "considerable" amount of home sewing to clothe yourself and your family. As well as comfort and warmth, your clothes were expected to supply you with sufficient decency to allow those associating with you to maintain their self-respect. Additionally, you were expected to set aside between a third and a half of the cost of garment replacements each year.

Single men required the same clothing as married men but made more frequent replacements as they did not have a spouse to take care of clothing maintenance for them. Single working women required a wardrobe of high-quality streetwear while married women relied on practical housedresses.

Table 3: Comparison of Annual Household Clothing Budgets 1920

Income	1 person	2	3	4	5
$780	20%	-	-	-	-
$900	20.23%	-	-	-	-
$1,200	16.75%	13%	14%	15%	15%
$1,800	16.67%	13.33%	13.33%	14%	14.67%
$2,400	-	11%	12.5%	14%	15%
$3,000	-	12%	13.2%	14.4%	15.6%
$5,000	-	10.8%	12%	13.2%	14.4%

Womenswear

Key Looks

The common perception of the smoking, dancing "Flapper", with her slim body clothed in a short, dropped-waist sack dress, wrapped in fur and bobbed hair covered by a cloche hat has become synonymous with the era. However, it was an attitude not a style of dress. Adopting the look was simply a matter of fashion, similar to today's skinny jeans.

It was a girl's anti-establishmentarian youth culture, cutting her hair to mimic the poor and wearing boyish clothes to look independent. The ideal body was boyish, slim and tanned. For some this required an elastic corset to smooth out breasts and hips, and a number of dietary fads. Tans became indicators of leisure and good health, and this led to shorter, sleeveless gowns with lower backs.

Clothing was much shorter and simpler in line than previously, in part due to First World War fabric shortages. These comfortable clothes also drew against the slacks women wore in factories and the need for dancing dresses that allowed a greater range of movement for exotic new dances like the Tango. Additionally, the involvement of artists, particularly the Avant Garde, resulted in block coloured clothing that was beautiful as well as practical.

It drew against the bright colour palette and fluid shapes of traditional Asian, African and South American clothing such as tunics, harem pants and kimono sleeves, and were enhanced with beading, embroideries in Egyptian and Russian motifs, tassels and fur or feather trims.

Generally daywear was dark and conservative. Working women bought fashionable clothing silhouettes in long lasting dark neutral colours, and seasonal (cheaper) accessories such as hats, gloves scarves and bags in the brighter colours. As early as 1921, it was noted that the streets were filled with crowds of black-clad women, so it is likely that black was the colour of choice for working class women at that time.

In contrast, eveningwear was bright.

Key Figures

Zelda Sayre, (future wife of F. Scott Fitzgerald) was the iconic sex, drugs, and Charleston flapper. Other daring dressers included dancer Josephine Baker with strategically placed adornments and actress Louise Brooks' low cut revealing gowns.

Key Designers

The silhouette "sack" dress referred to the ease of dressing without assistance though this had been evolving in the work of Paul Poiret (still going strong though his heyday had passed) and his straight empire line silhouettes as early as 1907.

Gabrielle "Coco" Chanel developed a line of "poverty chic" fashions reinterpreting the functional and comfortable clothing worn by working class people in luxury jersey fabrics. Her clothes included pants and short loose sheaths with dropped waists and straight hips. She also used plain, unfussy materials like military fabrics, and borrowed pockets and lapels from menswear.

Jean Patou became the father of sportswear with tennis skirts, knitted swimwear and knitwear designed to show off a sporty physique. Additionally, neckwear, fragrances and suntan oil. His store contained different rooms dedicated to each sport; horse riding, tennis, swimming, golf and aviation. He was the first designer to embellish clothes with his initials.

CHAPTER 4

1930s

THE 1930S WERE A SPLIT personality decade of personal security seeking thriftiness and Hollywood-driven "Golden Age of Glamour".

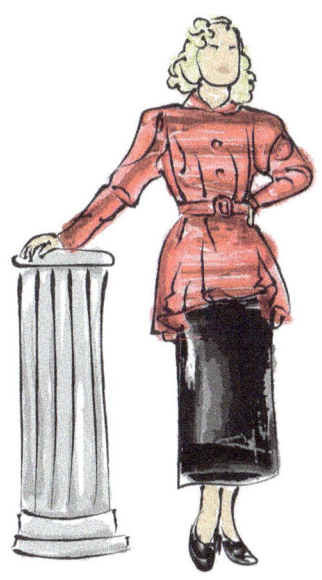

On the World Stage

Politics

During the 1930s, the League of Nations collapsed as many countries withdrew their membership. The Soviet Union collectivised agriculture and industry, and Stalin purged the "Old Bolsheviks" from the Communist Party. The Nazi Party took power in Germany, followed by German and Italian territorial expansion. The Irish rejected King George V and became a Republic with a new Constitution.

The Great Depression adversely impacted social, economic and political relationships across the globe, and so the decade was marked by high unemployment and poverty, with many governments launching work projects. Roosevelt was elected US President and launched the New Deal welfare strategy to combat the Depression. Canada gained Parliamentary independence, and Newfoundland returned to British rule. The US Board of Temperance Strategy was founded to fight the repeal of prohibition (which ended in 1933).

War

Like the previous decades, the 1930s had its share of large conflicts including the Chinese and Spanish Civil Wars, the Columbia-Peru, Chaco, Second Sino-Chinese and ongoing Castellammarese Wars. Not to mention the Second World War commencing in 1939. There was rebellion in India (resulting in limited self-governance) and China.

Disaster

In the US there was drought, dust storms and hurricanes. In China there were floods. The Hindenburg airship crashed and a gas leak caused an explosion and the destruction of a Texas school.

Science and Technology

Scientific and technological developments include the invention of Radio Directional Finding (Radar), Scotch Tape, nuclear fission and wide band frequency modulation radio as well as steam locomotive speed records.

Domestic Developments

Domestic developments include the first sales of Birdseye frozen foods, canned food, packaged cereals, the chocolate chip cookie and the wider availability of fresh produce. Also trans-Atlantic air mail services, the long-playing phonograph record, Kodachrome colour photography film, high definition television, the Volkswagen Beetle, commercial intercontinental flights, electric lap steel and bass guitars.

The Arts

Jazz music begins to make way for Swing and Blues.

Books included *The Hobbit*, *Brave New World*, *Grapes of Wrath*, *As I Lay Dying*, and *The Postman Always Rings Twice*. Along with the invention of comic book superheroes Superman and Batman.

Popular films include *Snow White and the Seven Dwarfs*, *Gone with the Wind* and *The Wizard of Oz*, as well as new horror features including *Dracula*, *Frankenstein*, *The Mummy* and *King Kong*. The first colour talking cartoon *Fiddlesticks* and the first widescreen *Song of the Flame*.

Art movements included Social Realism (Gropper), Mexican Muralism (Rivera), Bauhaus (Klee) and Dada (Picabla).

In Other News

Amelia Earhart disappeared during an attempt to circumnavigate the planet.

Social and Technological Developments in Fashion

Social Expectations

Partly driven by Hollywood, clothing was stylish despite being less expensive. Paris fashion remained influential, but American people were encouraged to buy local goods and import taxes were increased to ensure compliance (though some US citizens removed the labels to avoid paying the taxes). Additionally, department stores "clubbed" together to purchase models or relied on press photography. Some couturiers cut their costs by creating simpler clothing that required less fabric and labour, or introduced a "semi-couture" range with fewer fittings, or increased their use of synthetics.

Hollywood encouraged audiences to bond with its stars by giving young artists new personas with names and histories, "their" personalities portrayed consistently across all their movies, as well as in off-screen appearances. These iconic "people" became the ideal marketing tools and their movies large scale fashion shoots. Women were encouraged to imitate their favourite stars' dress, makeup and manners in order to achieve happiness, and copies of dresses and hats featured in movies were readily available.

Clothing became less formal and more practical - less restrictive and ornamented. As central heating and transport by car became more widespread, the need for heavy warm clothes like woollen underwear reduced. Hats and shoes became less important as status markers.

As well as comfortable and durable, daywear was now expected to be elegant, and consequently velvet became fashionable. Additionally, designers began using cotton and linen instead of silk in response to the need for less expensive clothing. The wealthy continued to purchase luxury fabrics, but artificial fibres gained in popularity over the period as cheaper alternatives. Fur remained in demand at a range of price points from mink down to rabbit to faux.

By the 1930s swimsuits were made from an elasticised fabric called Lastex that was knitted from cotton, wool or rayon covered rubber threads, which offered speed and fashion. The first sunscreen was released in 1936.

With the makeup and perfume markets expanding, new companies like Revlon and Elizabeth Arden began entering the market. The preferred look was natural, with pink ivory foundations, ivory mauve powders and sometimes pink blush with the newly invented lip gloss. As the decade progressed orange tinted foundations and darker lipsticks were popular. Eyebrows were plucked or shaved and then drawn back on in high dramatic arcs and glossed with Vaseline, as were dark smoky eyeshadows. The eyeshadow was chosen to match eye and hair colour as well as the outfit. Coloured nail polishes slowly grew in popularity, initially in pale pinks and as the decade progressed brighter and darker shades to coordinate with outfits, and lipstick. Makeup came to be seen as a luxury in times of hardship.

Advances in technology such as permanent waves and hot rollers changed the way women wore their hair with the smooth sleek bob transforming into fuller waves and curls. By 1932, the process of permanent waving had been reduced to a shorter chemical only process, with improved curly hair results. New safer dyes and Hollywood bombshells led the peroxide blonde trend.

As you might expect, families economised on presentation when times were tough, including less frequent haircuts and styles, replacing razor blades less frequently, and using washable sanitary supplies in preference to disposables.

Fabric Developments

Nylon, a synthetic polyamide fibre manufactured from chemicals, was invented in 1938 as an offshoot of work on a fibre that would become polyester. Its initial commercial success was interrupted by the Second World War when it was almost exclusively used for war matériel such as parachutes. It is strong, stretches, and recovers from stretching well making it perfect for hosiery, sheer fabrics and luggage.

Also during the late 1930s (in the lead-up to the Second World War), a number of economies took place in clothing manufacture, for example, rayon or cotton was blended with wool to produce cheaper fabrics. Similarly, silk was blended with or displaced by rayon. Additional fabrics were manufactured using lower grades of fibres, reduced thread counts and lighter threads. As more cotton was diverted to war production, rayon took a greater place in civilian dress. Other cost cutting methods included a greater reliance on machine manufacturing of things like collars and button holes, and reducing the use of more expensive materials for example, producing narrower hat bands.

Sewing Machines

As clothing costs escalated during the 1930s, quick and easy home sewing on new electric machines experienced a resurgence. Machines with full rotary gears, horizontal bobbins, improved gear rotation and bearings resulted in smoother operation. As the Depression and the US mass migration west and south-west continued, basic lightweight machines (in carry cases) were popular.

Manufacturing

Many more women were able to secure employment, and this led to a greater demand for ready-to-wear clothing and expansion of the industry. It also became common to wear ensembles of matching skirt and jacket (skirt suit), dress and jacket (dress suit) or skirt and blouse (two piece dress) over the usual single dress. The period also saw a move towards timeless classic "investment pieces".

Home sewing did not produce significant cost savings, so ready-to-wear clothes for women and children became more common, and the transition to factory clothing was almost complete. Despite this, many working class families did not have adequate clothing, and this did function as a status marker preventing full participation in the wider community.

The significance of their awareness of the new social norms is demonstrated by an increased expenditure on silk stockings. Women preferred to wear mended silk stockings with an old dress rather than a new dress without stockings.

The increase in magazine availability and sponsored content led to an increase in demand and consequently an explosion of ready-to-wear companies, particularly catalogue companies such as Sears and Littlewoods.

Good fit became more important as the decade progressed, and to meet this need Sears started selling "semi-made" clothing which was mostly finished with just the final fitting to be completed by the home seamstress. This captured women downgrading from made-to-measure to ready-to-wear, particularly those who were inexperienced sewers and/or were forced into the job market with little time to shop.

At this time, zippers were common in luggage, but around 1934 when the Royals started wearing them to fasten their pants, their popularity in clothing grew. Many men preferred button flies through to the end of the Second World War.

Meanwhile at Home

By the middle of the Depression, almost everyone in large cities had access to utility services, though there were still economic and regional differences. Householders purchased appliances such as stoves that provided the fullest immediate benefit first.

Housing

Home ownership increased, but more families were renting apartments. Housing, fuel and lighting costs increased. Generally, a single family lived in a five roomed home with electricity and gas, and a coal-fired stove or furnace for heat. Some houses would have been shared, needed major repairs or may have even been derelict. Additional problems included pests, inadequate ventilation and sunlight, and lack of privacy.

The major class differences were in things like refrigerators, clothes washing machines, central heating and telephones. Poor families wanted the basics (like windows), but the most affluent looked for luxuries like electrical outlets.

Water Supply

While there were still unplumbed homes, 90% had a full bath, and 80% hot running water. They were more comfortable with plumbing, bathrooms, heating, lighting and furnishings.

Doing the Laundry

Laundry still took time and effort, but smaller families and less structured clothing along with electric or gasoline washing machines made the task less onerous. The machines still required physical assistance for filling, wringing and changing the cycles. Up to 26% of working class households and 37% of the middle class bought assistance with the laundry.

Gas Supply

Gas cooking and central heating was becoming common.

Electricity Supply

Technological changes between the First World War and the Depression made the greatest impact on household drudgery including electric lighting, clothes washers, hot water heaters, refrigerators, stoves, vacuum cleaners, toasters, sewing machines, percolators and central heating despite their high cost. In 1934 - 35, 65% of homes relied on iceboxes, with only 28% having electric or mechanical refrigerators. Around 75% of homes had radios, a major source of entertainment and communication, some had two.

Telephone

While telephone service was a luxury and an indicator of status, about a quarter of working class families had one.

INCOME AND CLOTHING EXPENDITURE

Income

Those who lost jobs, or were in intermittent work fared the worst, but families with working husbands were generally not significantly affected by the Great Depression. Some sectors such as manufacturing were affected more than others, mainly through a reduction in work hours.

Income varied enormously across all classes depending on access to income support, and what income could be scraped up from elsewhere. Government income support came in the form of cash, work, or in-kind such as food, clothing or shelter depending on where you lived. It was difficult to access, and families who did were regarded as deviant and were not offered a path back to normality.

Many men set up their own businesses when they lost their jobs. Women moved from farm work to clerical, or employment in private homes. Teenaged girls spent longer at school and did not find work until later in life. Income from lodgers became more important than gifts.

The average 1935 total household income (from all sources) was:

- Working Class: $1,071
- Middle Class: $1,355
- Upper Class: $2,260

Clothing Expenditure

UK company Littlewoods started encouraging its customers to set up shilling clubs, a kind of group layaway arrangement in which participants contributed a shilling a week towards their purchases. When the club was set up a ballot was taken to determine the delivery order, and as Littlewoods received the money they sent the clothes in that order. All but the last received their order before it was paid for.

By 1935, the majority of working class UK families were "saving" for new clothes through clubs rather than buying second hand, and in 1939 this was about 3.5% of their income.

Around this time, weekly clothing expenses formed 51% of unexpected purchases despite a budget range of 8.1% to 33.3%. Budgets varied between 12.73% and 19.44% depending on the number and employment status of the children.

Even as incomes fell, families attempted to maintain their level of spending, to as much as 9% more than they earned. They drew from their savings, cashed in their insurance policies and/or entered credit arrangements.

Men spent a little less on clothing, and women spent correspondingly more. Many working class families had sufficient clothes for survival, but not enough for a social life. In the working class, cleanliness and repair became status markers, whereas the middle class bought more variety and quality.

While women still bought makeup, manicure supplies, a comb, toothbrush and deodorant, they did cut back on face powder, manicures and hairpins. Men bought a hairbrush and comb, shaving supplies, and toothbrushes for personal grooming, but used their razor blades until they were blunt enough to cause rashes, cuts and unevenness.

Unemployed families would have focused on men's presentation, with women and children cutting their hair at home.

Womenswear

Key Looks

During the Thirties, women's fashion grew up. The square flat silhouettes of the twenties grew longer hems, waistlines dropped further, then rose back to natural. Clothes began to hug the figure more closely with empire line jackets, and hip interest provided by yokes, layers and pleats. These produced the refined and glamorous sophisticated womanly silhouette we now see as quintessentially Thirties - curvy women in calf length dress and permed bob.

As the decade progressed clothing remained glamorous but as the likelihood of war and the need for functionality increased, nationalistic and military style elements with lower heels became more common. The Art Deco expressed positivism through bright colours and playful narrative prints that were particularly popular as conversational prints and as propaganda scarves during the war.

The comfortable sportswear trend still existed but became more feminine in keeping with the fashionable silhouettes of the time and more durable and practical as fabric technology changed. Some items such as swimsuits developed fashions of their own while others such as pyjamas found new life as beachwear.

Two-tone shoes like the "Spectator" became available for the first time, and as the depression deepened wedge shoes became common as a way to reduce the cost of shoe manufacture. Durable and practical leather bags replaced the Twenties beaded and enamelled ones. Hats were still seen as necessary, but the shapes became softer and more feminine to accommodate the fuller, more glamorous hairstyles of the period.

Key Figures

Clothing started to take on aspects of individual self-expression with ease and comfort, bias cutting and aspects of men's suiting. There were many looks to emulate:

- Amelia Earhart's boyish athleticism in jumpsuits and leather jackets

- Eleanor Roosevelt's anti-fashion

- Pancho Barnes (Florence Lowe) in menswear

- Marlene Dietrich's tuxedo and fedora, and black and white colour scheme

- Frida Kahlo's bright colours, feminine folk clothing and exaggerated facial hair

Key Designers

Madeleine Vionnet's bias cut fluid fabric drapes, cowl necks and halter tops became the template for the thirties look.

Elsa Schiaparelli added a shoulder focus with tailored jackets, puffed sleeves and dress clips to bring the focus up. This was also highlighted with lower necklines, ruffles, yokes and corsages. She developed wrap dresses, used visible zips, novelty buttons and bright colours. She worked with the Surrealist artist Salvador Dali and collaborated on designs like the "Tears Dress" that appeared torn showing the flesh underneath. Her knitwear featured trompe l'oeil images.

Mainboucher created slim athletic forms with wasp waists and boned strapless bodices. Many Hollywood costume designers also moved into retail with shapes, forms and details that expressed character. Gilbert Adrian brought subtle filmic touches whereas Travis Banton went big and theatrical.

CHAPTER 5

1940s

OFTEN SEEN AS A DECADE of austerity, the warring 1940s embodied the notion of noble self-sacrifice to overthrow evil.

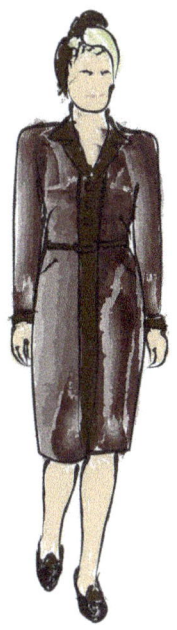

On the World Stage

War

Aside from the Second World War, there were a number of other conflicts during the 1940s, including the Arab-Israeli War, Greek and Chinese civil wars (resulting in the establishment of the People's Republic of China). Iceland separated from Denmark, Indonesia from the Netherlands, Syria and Lebanon gained independence from the French, and India, Pakistan, and Burma from the British. The United Nations and the North Atlantic Treaty Organisation (NATO) was established.

Science and Technology

Scientific and technological developments included nuclear physics, quantum and game theories, hydraulic fracturing and radiocarbon dating. Additionally assorted munitions, war matériels and technologies including jeeps, jet aircraft and the first digital computing devices.

Domestic Developments

Domestic developments included commercial television, the slinky, the frisbee, microwave ovens, Tupperware and velcro.

The Arts

Popular music styles were swing, the crooners (like Frank Sinatra), bebop and early rock and roll. Popular books were *For Whom the Bell Tolls*, *The Stranger*, *Pippi Longstocking*, *The Diary of Anne Frank* and *Nineteen Eighty-Four*. Popular films included *Mrs Miniver*, *Casablanca*, *The Maltese Falcon*, *It's a Wonderful Life*, *Citizen Kane*, *Great Expectations*, *The Red Shoes*, *Pinocchio*, *Dumbo* and *Bambi*. Art movements included

Abstract Expressionism (Pollock and de Kooning) and Fantastic Realism (Brauer and Fuchs).

In Other News

Thor Heyerdahl crossed the Pacific Ocean in the Kon-Tiki.

SOCIAL AND TECHNOLOGICAL DEVELOPMENTS IN FASHION

Social Expectations

As in the First World War, the best quality fabrics were set aside for military purposes leading to shortages and lower quality. Additionally, rationing took place across Europe and the US with associated austerity rules, and this froze the fashionable silhouette with only the details changing.

In the UK, about a quarter of the population was entitled to wear a uniform, and as this demand put pressure on manufacturing, battledress became the standard issue. Large numbers of women served in Auxiliary services; they did not see combat, but undertook a range of administrative, hospitality and driving tasks that would free up the men to perform more valuable war work (like fighting). Their uniform issue included otherwise difficult to obtain clothing.

Pants became less shocking as women wore them more often, particularly for their war work. Additionally, they were comfortable to wear and hid stockingless legs. Coats were generally masculine boxy affairs with large pockets, but capes and reversible raincoats were popular too. Fur was not rationed, so small touches like collars and cuffs brought a little glamour and femininity to otherwise utilitarian outerwear.

In the US, cars became more common as more families moved to less formal outer suburbs. Driving women commonly wore easy-care pants or shorts with blouses or shirts rather than the simple house dresses worn previously.

Eveningwear lost much of its formality, long gowns were replaced by long skirts with fitted blouses, and pieces such as embroidered jackets that worked for the afternoon as well as evening. That level of formality is now reserved for events, and no longer considered a general requirement for things like going out to a restaurant for dinner.

Hats took the tedium out of rationing, with a wide variety of styles available. Turbans were very popular, particularly as the war progressed and soaps were more difficult to obtain. Bags were larger, squarer, and more practical for carrying supplies to air-raid shelters, particularly satchels in circumstances when running might be required. With shortages of zippers and leather, drawstrings and plastics became popular, but after the war women preferred small ladylike leather bags.

Shoes made from rationed materials were expensive, so cheaper shoes with wood or cork soles and plastic and reptile skin uppers became common. The most popular styles were wedges, chunky heeled sling backs and Mary Janes or low heeled oxfords.

Swimwear continued to evolve with the Jantzen company introducing shorts and shirts to be worn over the top of swimsuits. During the decade, one piece swimsuits fell out of favour.

Makeup was not rationed during the war for fear of low morale, but it was very expensive. Women did not want to appear showy, but they did want to look and feel polished. In the UK, they found ways around shortages such as beetroot lipstick, boot polish mascara and gravy browning stockings. By 1946 permanent wave technology had developed to the point that it was available as a home treatment.

Fabric Developments

In the 1940s, silk was unavailable and rayon was in demand for stockings despite their tendency to sag and bag. After the Second World War, nylon's superior performance saw the end of rayon stockings and made nylon synonymous with stocking due to its low cost, high strength, stretch and durability.

The bulk of fabric dyes were reserved for military use resulting in a small colour palette for civilian clothing of browns, blues, greys and greens The Utility style directives promoted less waste which encouraged smaller scale patterns that could be more easily and efficiently matched at seams.

Synthetic and manufactured fibres were readily accepted after the Second World War for their advertised "easy-care", "drip dry" and "wash and wear" properties. Manufacturers added finishes that made them "permanent press", "wrinkle resistant" and "stain resistant". They also blended synthetics like polyester with natural fibres such as cotton to produce clothing that combined the comfort of natural fibres with the easy care of synthetics. Improvements in washing machine technology may also have increased uptake of synthetics.

Olefins like polypropylene and polyethylene were used in 1949 for non-textile uses but have now grown to include disposable nappies (diapers), sportswear (due to its excellent wicking properties), clean suits and protective clothing.

Modacrylic was introduced in 1949 (as Dynel). While it is weak, it is flame retardant, maintains its shape and can be texturized. It is common in fleece, pile fabrics and faux furs.

Sewing Machines

Emerging from the Depression, home dressmaking was still customary. Lightweight machine technology progressed with a 16 lb (7.25kg) machine.

By the Second World War, most sewing machine factories were commandeered to manufacture things like technical instruments and precision war tools like bomb sights and firing pins. The US War Production Board permitted some manufacture of sewing machines and parts, but regulated their sale, and this led to a thriving market in rental machines.

Post-war, new machines were on quota, with a long waiting list, though improvements like a free arm for mending things like pant legs, sleeves and socks continued.

Manufacturing

In an attempt to ensure good quality clothing was fairly accessible by all, the UK government introduced the Utility Scheme in 1942. It offered well designed, good quality and (most importantly) price controlled clothing that had to pass value for coupon tests for shrinkage, colour fastness and waterproofing.

It was one of a number of Utility manufacturing programmes, and unpopular until fashion designers including Edward Molyneux, Hardy Amies and Charles Creed were invited to design clothing for the scheme.

Another austerity measure was the imposition of standard clothing designs, including directives on the amount of fabric that could be used. These controlled things like the number and size of pockets and buttons, the width of seams, pleats and sleeves, and the amount of embellishment.

The scheme introduced high-end designers to mass market production and allowed standardisation of materials and processes that also increased efficiency.

It was supported by the 1942 Conservation Scheme which provided approval for a limited number of manufacturers to continue clothing production.

King George VI set an example by continuing to wear his pre-war suits, having his clothes patched and mended, and ensuring his family did not exceed their rations.

During the 1940s, a knitting process known as warp knitting was perfected. There are three kinds of machine that produce a different kind of knit:

1. Tricot (the most common) uses a compound needle with a secure connection to tricot bars. Two bar tricot is used for underwear and three or four for dresses and suiting. One bar is most often used to attach or bond linings. Tricots are also used for fabrics with floating threads like satin where the back surface can be brushed or treated to create a lace-like appearance.

2. Simplex is similar but produces a thicker fabric such as faux suede for bags and gloves.

3. Raschel knits appear more woven and result in simulated embroidery and faux-furs.

Meanwhile at Home

Housing

By 1946, US families considered their homes so private that they would not share it with others unless their circumstances were very dire, and then only as a temporary measure. The home had plumbing, heating, bathroom, kitchen, as well as a living room and the appropriate number of bedrooms; generally five rooms plus bathroom with sink, toilet, bath and/or shower. It was cheaper to buy than rent a home. Only the very poorest still rely on pumps, share toilets (in some cases still earth closets), and/or use fireplaces for heating and cooking.

Water Supply

In some cases, particularly in rural areas, households did not yet have running water, but city dweller's basic expectation was for clean hot and cold running water.

Doing the Laundry

As mains power spread it changed how chores were undertaken - transferring laundry work from a copper in the outhouse, to the porch in a washing machine, to an enclosed room with internal plumbing.

As the homemaker, the mother cooked, cleaned and washed the clothes and linens - she didn't have outside help but used appliances to help manage the physical strain.

After the war, manufacturers started encouraging upgrades to fully automatic washing machines that filled, washed, rinsed, spun dry and shut down. These machines eliminated wringer injuries and mishaps (tears and lost buttons), so laundry started to become a daily rather than weekly chore.

Gas Supply

By 1941, gas was increasingly replacing coal for cooking but its use for lighting was decreasing.

Electricity Supply

Electricity had become the most common source of power for lighting and appliances. Some homes still relied on generators, but the general expectation was electric lighting, central heating and hot water heater with tank storage.

Essential appliances (worth significant sacrifice to obtain) included gas or electric stoves, mechanical refrigerator (as opposed to ice box) and washing machine along with the power and plumbed water to use them. Others include iron, vacuum cleaner, toaster, and waffle iron.

Telephone

Many homes had phones but they were not thought essential.

INCOME AND CLOTHING EXPENDITURE

Income

The 1940s present a number of issues in determining income and expenditure, mainly due to the regulation of income, prices and production. Additionally, the majority of surveying was undertaken for war purposes so a lot of households were excluded from the data gathering.

However, people who enlisted or worked got paid, though there wasn't a great deal you could buy and what you could was expensive. The median wage in 1945 was:

- Working Class: $1,532
- Middle Class: $2,039
- Upper Class: $2,768

Clothing Expenditure

Clothing rationing was introduced in the UK in June 1941 to constrain civilian demand and to ensure fair distribution. Each garment was allocated a points value, but new clothes required both cash *and* coupons. The initial adult allocation was 66 coupons per annum, but by September 1945 this had fallen to 24. Each category of garment required the same number of coupons regardless of outlet such that an eight coupon shirt bought by the working class may have been less durable than an eight coupon shirt bought by the upper class from a high-end store.

With shortages increasing and coupons reducing, in 1943 women were urged to "Make Do and Mend" as a way to give something back to the war effort and take pride in self-sacrifice (as well as feel guilty for not doing as much as possible). A character called "Mrs Sew and Sew" was created to promote the scheme and give tips.

Classes and information were provided on clothing care, repair, making, remaking, repurposing and using unrationed fabrics such as blackout material and old blankets to make clothes as well as knitting and darning. Other initiatives included a children's clothing exchange.

The campaign was not well received by all as many had been making do for some time before the campaign launch. Some had been doing it so tough that they couldn't afford to buy or make clothes, and were selling their coupons on the black market for cash or food.

In the UK, rationing continued until 1949, and the Utility Scheme to 1952 but in the US rationing ended in 1946.

Womenswear

Key Looks

In the US, the key looks were optimistic romantic moralist power silhouettes:

- strong but sexy like "Rosie the Riveter"
- idealised and overtly sexy like Alberto Varga's pinup girls.

Pre-war American fashions took on a folk element, drawing initially against smocked and embroidered German folk costumes, but as the decade progressed against Latin American, cowboy and pioneer influences.

The UK Utility Scheme and design directives resulted in a look that was stable throughout the war: straight skirts with knee-length hems, jackets with broad shoulders, tapered waists and narrow hips forming an inverted triangle shape. These were showcased in close fitted day dresses, high waisted pants, blouses with bow ties and masculine tailoring or military style detailing - comfort and practicality were popular. While the silhouettes were stable, the decorative details were variable and used for individual expression. These were accented by red lipstick and platform shoes.

Key Figures

Hollywood movies adopted styles worn by "real" women; like Joan Crawford's self-sufficient ball busting career women or Rita Hayworth's rejection of fantasy lifestyles. Actresses like Katharine Hepburn made films with propaganda messages while Marlene Dietrich raised war bonds and toured with the United Service Organizations Shows. Hollywood stars were pictured in plain serviceable clothes doing their bit for the war effort, and many fashion shoots took place against backdrops of industry or airstrip.

Key Designers

US and UK designers were required to ensure their looks remained as fashionable for as long as possible so the lines and colours remained quite stable. Fabrics included wool and tweed, and looks included skirt suits, dresses that transitioned day to evening, button down and shirtwaist dresses, twin sets, box coats and knitwear. Separates were popular as they permitted a variety of looks from within a limited wardrobe.

Meanwhile in the US, lack of access to Parisian fashion combined with an excess of production capacity forced the local industry to come up with its own designs, and a rivalry between Los Angeles and New York as the fashion capital commenced. Movie designers like Adrian with their established reputations were ideally situated to take advantage of this gap in the market.

A national look of smart casual daywear and Hollywood style eveningwear was in development, helped along by Clair McCardell and Hattie Carnegie. These designers were reinterpreted and publicised by the Sears Roebuck catalogues to produce a range of practical fashions. McCardell brought sportswear into the office with the opinion that the role of clothes was to prepare women to live their best lives while Carnegie made clothes that brought the focus to the wearer not the garment for a kind of elegant everyday stylishness.

Despite Hitler's desire to shut down the couture industry and transfer it to Berlin, many Paris fashion houses reopened or remained open during the war under threat of Nazi confiscation. The Germans imposed restrictions on the couturiers though these were not as harsh as those imposed in the UK.

Madame Gres (who sculpted evening gowns by draping vast swathes of silk around the body leaving little spaces where you might glimpse it) was among the designers the Nazis shut down for exceeding yardage, or "offensive" designs.

French fashions of the period reinterpreted the nineteenth-century fashions for bustled full skirts, lush embellishments and tall hats, and these seemed very shocking to the liberating Allies with their backdrop of austerity.

They were scorned for a couple of years, the impasse only broken by a collection produced by new couturier Christian

Dior with a full skirted, soft shouldered and small waisted continuation of the nineteenth-century reinterpretation. He was financed by a fabric manufacturer who required that the designs use a luxurious amount of fabric. His designs brought eveningwear style into the daytime.

The New Look did not end the popularity of Utility Style, partly because garments could not be manufactured cheaply, partly due to political ridicule at the amount of waste embodied in the garments, and partly because it was seen as regressively hiding women's legs and impeding their movement.

American designers reinterpreted the look and reduced its formality by removing the boning and shortening the hems. There were also a number of "make do and mend" style tutorials on how to replicate the look by adding yokes.

CHAPTER 6

1950s

THE BOOMING 1950S BLENDED INDIVIDUALISM with a strong work ethic. Stability and suburban contentment were at odds with the civil rights movement and the cold war.

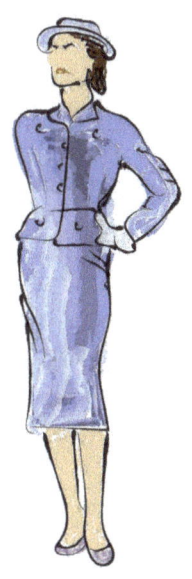

ON THE WORLD STAGE

Politics

During the 1950s, the European Common Market was established, though Europe remained Western and Soviet Bloc divided by the Iron Curtain and the Berlin Wall (dividing the Western Federal Republic of Germany from the communist German Democratic Republic). Alaska and Hawaii joined the United States and the North American Aerospace Defence Command (NORAD) was established.

War

The end of the Second World War, led into the "Cold War"; a standoff between the United States and the United Soviet Socialist Republics. It became a de facto war against Communism involving conflicts in Korea, Vietnam and Cuba. The Arab-Israeli conflict continued, Algeria fought and won independence from France, and the African Hutu/Tutsi conflict began. US troops withdrew from Japan, leaving it an independent nation once again. France granted independence to Laos, Cambodia and Vietnam. General Gamal Abdel Nasser Hussein overthrew the Egyptian monarchy later becoming its President. There were large scale decolonisation of African nations including Libya, Sudan, Morocco, Tunisia and Ghana.

Disaster

There were earthquakes in India and Algeria, floods in India, Uruguay, the Netherlands and the UK, volcano eruptions in Papua New Guinea, hurricanes in Haiti and the US, and a typhoon in Japan. Also a dam collapse in France, aeroplane crashes in the UK, Germany, Japan, the US, Italy and Ireland. The cruise liner SS Andrea Doria crashed into MS Stockholm and sank.

Science and Technology

In science and technology there was the invention of solar panels and a solar powered watch, sputnik and the Space Race followed by the establishment of the National Aeronautics and Space Administration (NASA), microwave amplification, more munitions, the polio vaccination, the double helix structure of Deoxyribonucleic Acid (DNA), medical ultrasounds and human trials of drugs like lysergic acid diethylamide (LSD) and chlorpromazine, as well as transorbital lobotomies. The Conseil Européen pour la Recherche Nucléaire (CERN) also known as the European Organization for Nuclear Research was established, as was the first nuclear power plant.

Domestic Developments

Domestically, almost all US homes had televisions, and they started getting bigger. President Truman made the first transcontinental television address. The first plastic Coca-Cola bottle was manufactured.

The Arts

Popular music was classic pop, rock and roll, folk and doo-wop.

Books included *The Catcher in the Rye*, *Lolita*, *Fahrenheit 451*, *Breakfast at Tiffany's*, *Lord of the Flies*, *Charlotte's Web*, and *The Tin Drum*.

Popular movies included *Ben-Hur*, *North by Northwest*, *Gentlemen Prefer Blondes*, *The African Queen*, and *The Ten Commandments* along with 3D pictures like *Man in the Dark*, and the debut of stereophonic sound in *House of Wax*.

Art movements included Colour Field Painting (Newman and Rothko) and Pop Art (Warhol).

Social and Technological Developments in Fashion

Social Expectations

The Depression, Second World War and subsequent legislation had set US working hours at eight hours a day, five days a week. The addition of paid vacation days and higher wages resulted in a great deal more leisure time. Reading and movies remained popular, but radios, photography, sports and toys were increasingly in demand.

Movies, magazines and television began creating a new market segment that came to be known as teenagers. They were working and had their own money to spend, and consequently fashion started to swing away from parents and towards them. Teenagers copied their film and music idols, settling into two competing groups the black leather and denim clad "greasers" and the neat and tidy "preppies'.

Everyday life was becoming less active, and exercising for fitness transforming into a leisure activity. Wealthier families could afford to purchase sporting equipment and clothing as well as club memberships. Social activities were a more important part of life, as were family outings and vacations. The ability to attend purchased events such as concerts or sporting matches were becoming status indicators.

With more social activities came a greater emphasis on personal appearance. Treatments at beauty and barber shops became part of social and recreational life. The way your hair looked was a marker of your social standing, and professional shampoos and permanent waves were an important way of indicating this. Hair was worn in soft pageboy waves, short curly (poodle) perms or up in chignons and French pleats. Home permanents and dyes became more common as the Clairol advertising slogan asked "Does she or doesn't she?" At the very least, working class women were expected to wear makeup and have clean and neatly styled hair.

Cosmetics and other toiletries now accounted for 10% of personal care expenditures (the first non-smear lipstick was invented in 1950). Makeup was heavy; pale face with rouged cheeks, high arched eyebrows, darkly lined eyes, coloured shadow and mascara, dark red lips.

Women still wore hats and gloves when they left the house.

Fabric Developments

In 1952, the first acrylic fibre was marketed under the name Orlon. It resembles wool and despite its weakness is used as a low-cost substitute.

In 1953, polyester was released in the US as Dacron and in the UK as Terylene. It is produced in different strengths and blends that affect its hand feel, but all are generally easy to launder. It was commonly found in pantsuits and was unpopular for a time due to low-quality fibres though it has become more popular recently with the introduction of microfibres.

Work jackets came in a new range of lightweight fabrics. Those with money to spend bought ventilated fabric; an open weave mix of wool fibres, but ready-to-wear came in Dacron, Orlon and Dralon (another acrylic fibre). They also came in wool blends that were light, kept their shape and remained wrinkle free though they were often unpleasant to wear and not well cut.

The elastomer, a polyurethane based synthetic rubber fibre was invented in 1959 under the name Lycra (also known as spandex and elastane). It is stronger than rubber with excellent elongation and recovery making it useful for sporting and underwear. It is quick drying, resistant to sun, sea water and chlorine, therefore, good for swimwear as well. More recently it has been incorporated in a wide range of fabrics to improve fit and comfort.

Sewing Machines

By the 1950s, the sewing machine had almost reached the level of technology at which we see it today. It had zig zag stitching, and in some machines a slanted needle made it easier to see what you were sewing. The stitch template discs were released. Some machines had darning and monogram capability, as well as twin-needles for decorative stitching.

Manufacturing

The economic and political events that took place after the Second World War saw the establishment of the conditions that would ultimately result in the outsourcing of clothing manufacturing.

America's post-war occupation of Japan was intended to help rebuild its political and industrial systems. Japan's textile industry was a major part of this work, partly because it had been one of the most globally competitive, particularly in cotton, silk and rayon, accounting for about 60% of its exports, and partly because it would not aid future aggression. The world's post-war economy wasn't liquid, so the US sold cotton to Japan and then bought it back as cheap fabric and clothing, which led to political difficulties when American unions and manufacturers opposed the imports.

As the cold war continued, similar interventions were used in Taiwan and South Korea to combat communism. As the communists took power in China, refugees brought the skill and capital required to set up manufacturing facilities in Hong Kong and Taiwan. Foreign Aid also assisted the creation of new facilities in Singapore, the Philippines, Pakistan and India, and the reduction of import tariffs made foreign manufactured clothing increasingly economical for consumers.

MEANWHILE AT HOME

Housing

In the US, home ownership increased rapidly during the 1940s as the government sold its rent controlled homes to their residents and it was still cheaper to own than rent a home. Across all classes families preferred new homes as they were larger, more modern, had gardens, were located in outer city suburbs and offered more control over the living environment. Renters tended to live in apartments in the city.

The average home consisted of four to six rooms for three residents, private toilet and bath, running water, central heating, gas or electric stove. As the cost of electricity was becoming cheaper than the cost of ice, iceboxes were replaced with mechanical refrigerators.

Locational differences in open space, easily accessible public transport, crime, noise, schools, hospitals, libraries and the like provided additional markers of status difference. Higher class homeowners were able to keep their homes in better repair than lower, for example, painting more frequently.

Water Supply

While there was some regional variation, only the very poorest lived in homes without running water - most had a private toilet and bath with hot running water.

Doing the Laundry

The increasing use of electric appliances such as washing machines took the drudgery out of laundry but set higher standards for clothing cleanliness. Hanging clothes out to dry remained the main labour, but many higher class families were also purchasing clothes dryers. About a third of families sent some laundry out.

Gas Supply

Fuel oil replaced coal as the most common source of energy though gas and electricity were more common as class increased. Wood was still in use, but more as a recreational than necessary source of energy.

Electricity Supply

The increasing use of electric appliances such as refrigerators set higher standards for the variety and freshness of food. Items also considered essential included vacuum cleaners, toasters and irons, with higher class families also purchasing freezers. Many of these larger items were bought with payment plan credit.

Appliance quality was becoming a status marker, higher classes spent more money on automatic washers while the lower classes spent less on non-automatic.

A third of homes had commercial television by the 1950s and three-quarters by 1956. It standardised culture across the US, and as programming focused on more affluent families, it served to stimulate demand for aspirational goods. Again, higher classes bought bigger and more attractive television sets.

Telephone

The telephone was cheaper and more common in homes across the classes, it had become the primary means of communication despite costing twice as much as postal services. Not having one led to some social exclusion.

INCOME AND CLOTHING EXPENDITURE

Income

At this time husbands and some wives worked for pay, but most children did not.

By 1950, the numbers of married women in the workforce had reached their highest level with many refusing to return to full-time home duties after the war. As educational participation increased, they replaced children as supplementary workers. Consequently, household income was 60% greater than 1935. The average gross household income in 1950 was:

- Working Class: $2,671
- Middle Class: $3,708
- Upper Class: $4,807

With higher incomes came greater community participation, and a comparable spread of expenditure across the classes.

Craft and operational jobs increased to 40% of the male labour market as farming and labouring jobs decreased, with an additional 13% in service occupations and 13% managerial.

Clothing Expenditure

All family members were becoming more fashion conscious and purchasing a wider range of clothing for work, social, leisure, sports and recreation.

As ready-to-wear clothing increased in quality and availability once more, clothing became less of a status marker, though each class developed its own distinctive version of simplicity. The higher classes were easily identified by their newer and more varied clothing as well as more expensive watches and coats while homemade clothes indicated lower status.

Clothing became less formal, with suits and dresses replaced by separates, though in general people owned the same number of street outfits as in 1935. Heavy woollen underwear was replaced by cotton as the availability of cars and central heating made extra warmth less necessary. The bulk of women's clothing budgets went on easy-care synthetic dresses and underwear like slips and bras, as well as nylon stockings.

The working class was spending 50% more on clothing than in 1935 though women of all classes spent more than men. They bought more clothes as the family's economic position increased, particularly teenage girls who now spent 60% of the cost of their mothers spend. Men spent less than previously, and young men generally spent 67% less than their fathers.

Clothing services like dry cleaning and shoe repairs accounted for 12% of the clothing budget.

WOMENSWEAR

Key Looks

Tired, ration-weary women were looking for feminine and elegant sophistication, with tailored suits, twin sets and shirtwaist dresses for the day, and cocktail dresses and evening gowns for evening. The two key looks were the hourglass shape with corsetry cinched waists and full petticoated skirts or the shapeless sack dress rebranded as the shift dress. Working women wore wool pencil skirt suits with silk blouses and stilettos.

While women were already wearing pants casually, the introduction of polyester led to pant suits becoming suitable business wear for women. However, some were of such low quality that "polyester pantsuit" became a derogatory term and pant suits fell out of favour though the pants themselves did not. Since then, the reduction in the fibre size (microfibre) has increased comfort and drape and popularised polyester once more.

Key Figures

The key archetypes in the fifties were the beautiful and untouchable Grace Kelly and the voluptuous and dominant Betty Paige. Or perhaps the Doris Day girl next door and sexy Elizabeth Taylor. But Mamie Eisenhower's cheerful and comfortable pink femininity with pearl chokers and charm bracelets probably more accurately represents how middle class American women really dressed.

Key Designers

Around this time, a number of developments took place including Bonnie Cashin's layered dressing (and boots as a fashion accessory), Anne Klein's junior sophisticates, Jacques Fath bringing attention back to the hips and bottom and Emilio Schuberth's strapless, ultra feminine lace confections.

Cristóbal Balenciaga was one of the key designers of the decade, taking inspiration from his Spanish homeland and deemphasising the waist, broadening the shoulders and increasing attention on the back. His key silhouettes include tunics, empire line, babydoll, column, shift and chemise dresses, as well as balloon jacket and cocoon coat.

A Chanel resurgence introduced soft jerseys in easy shapes and simple colours, which allowed women to dress without help (with zippers and so on). These were accessorised with bold costume jewellery statement accessories. She created the simple everyday style of braided suit with gold chains and white blouse. Other touches included monogrammed buttons and quilted bags on chains.

After meeting to develop costumes for the movie *Sabrina*, Hubert de Givenchy (then an unknown couturier) and Audrey Hepburn (unknown actress) became the first designer/star partnership, in a relationship that spanned more than 40 years. He is best known for developing lines of separates, and luxury ready-to-wear collections.

Italian designers became more influential in fashion. Emilio Pucci for trouser suits and shift dresses and bold swirling abstract prints in acidic colours. Roberto Capucci for dramatic sculptural dresses.

PART TWO: Develop Your Wardrobe Plan

IF YOU WORK THROUGH THIS part step by step you will develop a wardrobe plan consisting of a set of purchasing principles to guide your shopping, and the start of your basic annual shopping list.

CHAPTER 7

Step 1: Set Your Budget

The most important place to start your wardrobe planning process is deciding how much you can spend. You might disagree with me, but putting a limit on your spending makes you think seriously about what you *need* versus what you *want*. More importantly, knowing what you can spend sets boundaries around the quantity and quality of items you can buy.

Of course putting together a wardrobe might not seem to be on the same scale of things that need a budget like buying a car or renovating your kitchen. But you wouldn't do either of those things without considering what you could afford, your purpose, colours and the features you want (like wear and tear or durability). And while the odd garment here and there doesn't seem like much, over the course of a year you could be spending the purchase price of a car or do-it-yourself kitchen makeover.

You don't need vast cash reserves to dress well, in fact having them might prevent you from dressing well because you can afford to buy the latest "it" thing regardless of whether it suits you or it goes with any other thing in your wardrobe. All you *need* is the right clothes, and they are the ones that are appropriate for your lifestyle, meet your style requirements and for preference work with your existing wardrobe.

Two people with the same budget may differ greatly in their opinion about its adequacy - one may think it a pittance and the other an overabundance. Regardless of your opinion about the adequacy of the amount, you *can* fit expensive designer clothes into a tight budget by carefully prioritising your purchases and looking for bargains.

How Much To Spend

In 1935, your *household* clothing budget was a proportion of household income. At the time, people weren't paying income tax, but these days most of us have it deducted from our salary before we receive it, so I suggest that you base your budget on your take home pay. They identified four levels of income:

- subsistence 10 - 12% (say living in poverty)
- minimum comfort 12 - 15% (working class)
- comfort 16 - 17% (middle class)
- liberal 18 - 20% (upper class)

A lot has changed in the last 80 years, for example, ready-to-wear clothing is cheaper because it is mass produced offshore in manufactured or synthetic fibres, so you are probably wondering whether these percentages are still useful.

In a 1928 study, a woman bought an everyday dress for $2 (expecting two years wear) and spent the same on a visit to a doctor. For me, that's about $80, and I could get a reasonably good quality dress that is practical and durable for $80 in which case the allocation seems valid.

However, an everyday outfit of track pants and a t-shirt at $25 to last a year would be $50 (for two years). In higher quality materials they would be more durable and last longer so $80 still looks about right.

On the other hand, jeans and a button down shirt takes the cost up to $200, and this outfit will last around two and a half years. So $80 is still sufficient.

Our 1928 woman would have changed clothes when leaving the house to run errands, and with an everyday outfit of track pants and t-shirt you should too. But with jeans and a button down, you could just smear on some lipstick and go so the cost of additional street clothes could be offset. The $80 allocation is still reasonable.

The majority of people will identify as working or middle class, and will fall within the 12 - 17% range. This gives you a little scope to pick where you think you fit. For example, if you were living in Australia at June 2015, and your annual salary was $50,000, your net income would be $42,203. This puts your annual clothing budget in the range of $5,064 - $6,330.

What to Include

An annual budget of $5,064 - $6,330 *does* sound like a lot, but might feel more manageable at $422 - $527.50 per month.

I've been calling it a "Clothing Budget", because as the statistical collection groups and methods changed, it became an amount just for clothing. Household linens moved into "Household Furnishings", and as the technologies changed, makeup and skin care joined hairdressing to become "Personal Care".

I include alterations, dry cleaning, jewellery and makeup in my clothing budget. My friend Katy just has clothes with a separate budget for her expensive brand name skin and hair care, makeup, hairdressing, facials and massage. Depending on how you feel about your budget number, you can decide what it covers.

Regardless of that, this is just a place to start - you can change it later because this process is all about you. But before you change it, pick an amount within your 12 - 17% range and work through the rest of the steps to see how it works. Then you will be in a better position to judge its adequacy.

How to Split It

If you live alone, congratulations - you get to spend all that money on yourself! Otherwise, you may have to share it, which leaves the question of how to split it fairly across all members of the household.

I say household, but the statistical assumption during this tie was that a household consisted of a nuclear family - husband (breadwinner, 38), wife (homemaker, 36), boy (13) and girl (8). Life is not as statistical and it's possible that you may be supporting parents and/or siblings as well as children. Some or all of these occupants may contribute some or all of their income to the household pot, and this may need to be factored into your clothing budget split.

Another thing to consider is that clothing budgets have always been fluidly responsive to circumstances; when times were tough, the proportion allocated to non-working wives went down based on the assumption they needed to leave the house less. The proportion allocated to husbands generally increased because they were the main sources of income and

Signature Wardrobe Planning

needed to be presentable for work. Allocations for children varied little though there was less new clothing coming in.

A number of proportion suggestions have been made over time, including:

- 30% husband (manual worker), 35% wife (office worker) and 35% for the statistical two children.

- 31% husband (working class), 25% wife (homemaker), 23% boy and 21% girl.

- 35% husband (middle class), 23% wife (homemaker), 22% boy and 20% girl.

You will need to adapt this for your particular circumstances, for example, if you:

- are a homemaker you might allocate yourself less.

- are a bread winning lawyer you might need a number of high-quality suits.

- are a care worker you might need a lot of easy-care clothes.

- have lots of kids you might want to allocate them a larger proportion, or less if you have hand-me-downs.

- have older kids you might want a new wardrobe for them to go to college with.

The variables are endless, but these should give you some ideas for determining the best scenario for you and your family. Be aware that this first year will probably not go to plan, and the more people that are covered by it, the more likely it is to go wrong. And that is perfectly fine; what you learn this year will make it easier for you to construct a better and more relevant wardrobe plan for next year. And what you learn next year will change your plan for the year after.

How to Get the Best Value

As I mentioned earlier, your budget sets limits on the number and quality of clothes you can buy.

You need to spend your money where you'll get the best value; that is, spend the most money on the clothes you'll wear most of the time.

Don't spend 90% of your money on clothes you'll only wear 2% of your time (Princess Clothes).

If you like timeless classics that might mean buying a $150 pair of leather flip flops you'll happily wear continuously for three years.

But if you like to dress more fashionably, you might prefer a $50 pair you can discard at the end of summer. Or perhaps five $10 pairs in different colours.

You can quantify value for money on a cost per wear basis. For example, if you wear your summer sandals all weekend for six months of the year, that's 52 wears. For that six months, the cost of each of those 52 wears is:

- $2.88 for the $150 pair
- $0.96 for the $50 pair
- $0.19 for the $10 pair.

If you calculate the $150 pair over two years, the cost per wear reduces to $1.44. And over three years, $0.96.

If you have a small budget you may be better off thrifting, or if you have a substantial budget perhaps you'll have clothes made-to-measure.

Somewhere in between but closer to bespoke you might go to high-end department stores or somewhere closer to thrift, big box stores.

Signature Wardrobe Planning

Advice on maximising value from 1937, provides some useful guidelines:

- base your wardrobe on one practical dark colour (e.g., blue, black or brown) and buy all your key items (coat, bags, shoes and dresses) in this colour.

- supplement with brighter blouses, jackets, scarves, belts and jewellery.

- buy clothes in simple silhouettes, fabrics and patterns that can be used for more than one season and/or purpose (e.g. work and social). Plain clothes provide an ordinary background for distinctive accessories and can be worn more often than easily recognisable clothes.

- buy clothes for who you are RIGHT NOW (your actual age, size, location and occupations) not who or what you want to be, or where you would like to go.

- buy your clothes from different stores at different price points - spend more on your everyday street clothes, and less on your house and leisurewear.

- "cheap" is not sufficient reason to buy clothes that don't fit well, have the wrong trim or care requirements you're not willing to fulfil.

- always remember that unworn clothes are a waste of money.

Some of the ways you might put this into practice include:

- buy one inexpensive simple evening dress in a practical colour and disguise it with contrasting accessories like statement jewellery or coloured jackets.

- buy plain, well-made underwear.

- only wear white in summer - it doesn't fade or go out of fashion. If you buy in natural fibres you can bleach them to keep them white.

- buy classics to last three to five years.

- keep pretty buttons and buckles from discarded clothes to replace less attractive ones.

- patch, mend and makeover clothes (you could use ribbons, lace or applique).

- buy staples (e.g. underwear and socks) on sale.

- shop at thrift, second-hand and consignment stores.

- if it's cheaper and you enjoy it, make your own clothes.

There are other kinds of value besides value for money. In the wardrobe context, there's the pleasure you get from looking for and buying items, researching, comparing prices and matching styles and colours to name a few.

My friend Toseland doesn't think a great deal about the clothes he buys, but when he's looking for computers, televisions or other appliances he compares features and benefits and chooses his purchases for other reasons than cost.

I can tell by the way he discusses his research he enjoys that more than the actual purchase. If you are this kind of shopper, then indulge yourself and schedule time to do it "properly".

On the other hand, if you're the kind of person that likes to shop for little treats as the year goes by, then acknowledge this and leave space in your budget for them rather than buying clothes without any clear intentions for them.

SUMMARY

Your clothing budget provides a framework for your spending:

- as a proportion of NET (after-tax) household income, and
- as a proportion of household expenditure reflecting your requirements.

Knowing your budget puts boundaries around your purchases and allows you to plan them with the best value in mind.

CHAPTER 8

Step 2: Determine Your Appropriate

Your signature wardrobe is built by you, especially for you. Each of the items in your closet should be chosen to support you to do the things that you do, in the places that you usually find yourself doing them. Generally this will be easy because you probably live in the same town, visit the same places and do the same things most of the time.

But it will also be incredibly difficult because you have probably just been buying what's available and not thinking deeply about the purpose, colours and features you need. Clothes chosen with this in mind will not only be a unique reflection of your environment and activities but give you confidence and make you comfortable wherever you find yourself.

If you do not decide what is appropriate, you are just buying random things from a bewildering array of shapes and styles and trends and fashions that may not be functional or practical for you.

Setting your budget automatically excludes some options; you either are or are not an haute couture shopper. Aside from that, there are some other issues you need to consider when you are determining whether a garment is appropriate for you.

Clothing Care

Your first decision has to be the time, effort and expense you are willing to put into maintaining your clothes.

Our $2 dress buyer from 1928 had limited clothing care options; she did not have running water or electricity to her house, so it's likely her family would have worn one set of clothing while the other was in the wash 1900 style. You, on the other hand, might wash every day because you can, or maybe once a month because you have to do your washing in a coin laundry in a bad part of town.

Aside from that:

- What is your tolerance for the number of wears in between washes? You might be comfortable washing your jeans after ten wears, but prefer to wash your t-shirts after every wear.

- Can you afford a lot of dry cleaning? While many clothes with dry clean only tags may not require this special care, items that are not colourfast, prone to shrinkage or are heavily embellished will. Simple clothes such as lined jackets might cost you $10, but a sequined evening dress requires gentle handling and will cost a great deal more. You will wear and clean your evening dress less often than your blazer, but if you don't want to pay someone to clean it, don't buy one with a dry clean only tag.

- Are you willing to hand wash your delicates? By delicates, I mean clothes made from fabrics like silk, lace and knitted wool. Hand washing isn't hard, and it doesn't take long, but it isn't something you can do while you are doing anything else. You must make the time and space available, and if you aren't willing to do that don't buy clothes with hand wash tags. (If you're not sure, there are some hand washing instructions in chapter 19 [Clothing Care]).

- Are you willing to iron? There is no doubt about it, ironing *is* one of the most tedious laundry tasks ever. On the bright side, it is something you can do while you are watching television, and might be the perfect excuse to stay home and catch up with *House of Cards*.

Make these care decisions your foundation purchasing principles; don't buy dry clean only, hand wash, do not tumble dry, and so on.

Climate

Where you live (most of the time) will affect what you wear.

For example, if you live in the tropics the temperature will be fairly constant throughout the year. You might not have "winter" but you probably have a monsoon season, when there is a high level of background humidity. You will be more comfortable wearing loose clothing that permits the free flow of air and encourages the evaporation of perspiration. Natural fibres are more effective at drawing perspiration from the skin and allowing it to evaporate than synthetics. However, wool and silk are excellent insulators so the best fabric choices will be cotton and linen. Additionally, lighter colours reflect more heat and will be cooler than dark. So the ideal tropical garment would be something like a loose white cotton shirt. You might also like a nice sun hat.

At the other end of the spectrum, if you live in the arctic you will have long cold winters and short cool summers. It will be more important for you to build up layers of clothing that trap warm air while drawing off perspiration and allowing your skin to breathe. Your first layer should probably be a long sleeved undershirt, long johns and warm long socks. As mentioned above, wool is an excellent insulator so this would be a good choice. Your middle layer is for insulating, and should be something that draws moisture away and might be something like a fleece tracksuit. The outer layer is more for protection from the wind and snow (not rain) and needs to breathe so something like quilted down would work well. You might need a microfibre balaclava and/or scarf, fur lined hat, thick mittens and insulated boots. You will want to avoid cotton as it doesn't easily release the moisture it absorbs, but you should consider technical synthetics such as Polartec for their quick dry properties.

Most of us of live somewhere in between these extremes, and will probably need some variation in our clothes for summer and winter. Our 1928 family had a definite seasonal focus, with a half summer half winter spend.

Think about how you feel in your summer and winter, and decide what clothes are appropriate for those conditions.

REGION

Similarly, your location in a city, rural or remote area will impact your purchasing decisions.

Take walking shoes for example; in the city you might just want a flat shoe that you can comfortably wear on asphalted streets between the train station and your office. In a rural region, you might be walking along rutted dirt tracks and need something more like an all-terrain shoe, and in remote areas something more like a hiking boot.

Your winter coat will require similar consideration - a cashmere wool coat is probably not durable enough for remote living, and a multi-pocketed mountain parka will look out of place in the city.

In the city, you are never far from a store and won't need a big bag, but in rural locations you might need to carry a wider range of items and need pockets that fasten and/or a large backpack.

Consider how your location affects your needs and make some decisions about what clothes and shoes are the most appropriate for them.

CAREER

What you do for a living also influences your purchases. Where your workwear is appropriately durable and of sufficient quality, it demonstrates your intelligence and good judgement. Of particular importance to women, it also sets boundaries and should, therefore, provide greater coverage than the clothes you wear with friends and family for more intimate occasions.

If you are a construction or other manual worker you need clothing that is durable and offers good protection such as jeans. You might need protective footwear with steel capped toes and perhaps gaiters for additional protection around the ankle and calves. Long sleeved shirts, thick gloves, hard hats and a tool belt all have their place in the wardrobe for this kind of worker. A wool blend skirt suit is not going to be practical for this line of work.

However, a good quality suit paired with discreet jewellery expresses a lawyer's professionalism and emotional distance from the matters at hand. Depending on their area of expertise they may also require prescribed court dress, and perhaps shiny shoes and a good quality briefcase or bag, but probably not a tool belt or a hard hat.

What clothes are the most appropriate for your work?

Leisure Activities

As with career, your out of office activities preclude some choices. Your Warcraft gaming clothes will probably be stretchy comfortable clothes that are good for a long hard sit, and possibly a character costume for conventions. However, for horse riding you will prefer jodhpurs, long sleeved shirts, riding boots, gaiters, a riding hat, gloves, jacket and possibly some sort of padded body protection. Perhaps costumes for jumping or dressage.

Your house clothes should also be appropriate for the activities at hand - not just your leisurewear, but all of it. Don't think that because others rarely see them they don't matter because they really do. Making the time and effort to dress well inspires your own confidence in yourself, your family's love and respect, and the admiration of friends and callers.

You should also make provision for at least one "good" outfit for church, concerts, parties and so on. That way, when an unexpected opportunity comes up, you will have *something* to wear. Your budget may not be big enough to have one outfit specifically for church, and one for the concert hall (and so on). But, you can afford one moderately expensive fashionable outfit that suits your style perfectly, which will work for all these activities when appropriately accessorised. It will make you feel good, and perhaps next year you might choose to buy another.

HEALTH

This won't be a concern for everyone, but it does make some choices unwise and potentially waste your precious clothing budget. If you have dodgy ankles you probably should't wear stilettos. If you're expecting some kind of surgery, you might want clothes that are loose and comfortable. Maybe you have scars you want to conceal, or are taking medication that is making you bloat. You get the picture.

PREGNANCY

Pregnancy is a dynamic time of body shape change that lasts for about six months, followed by further postnatal changes. It could change your clothing requirements for 12 months or more, so you might find it useful to put together your wardrobe plan on that basis. You will receive advice about this from everyone, so I'll keep it short and straightforward.

Fortunately for you, modern mothers have more options and fewer constraints than their early twentieth century counterparts, so you can focus on simplicity and comfort. Many of these items could take you through pre and post pregnancy if chosen well.

- Leggings will make you feel like a normal human being. You can buy maternity ones or size up in regular, and potentially wear them for some time after the birth. Or if that doesn't feel formal enough, some fold over waisted yoga pants, or *really* stretchy skinny jeans (the jeans probably should be maternity ones).

- Long loose tunics can be worn as a dress early on, with leggings as your pregnancy progresses, and maybe as a dress again after. If loose enough, it can also be used for discreet breastfeeding.

- Dresses in stretchy fabrics provide good bump coverage; it may be possible to size up in ordinary clothing rather than buying maternity.

- Loose unstructured cardigans that you can wrap around yourself. Thicker knits are more durable, can be worn as a light coat and will provide better nipple concealment (if that concerns you). Or if you need or want more formality, try a blazer. If you don't gain too much extra weight across your back and arms you may be able to wear one you already own.

- The most wonderfully beautiful scarf that you can afford, something amazing that you can wear when you don't want to wear the same old thing yet again. You can use it as a wrap, or knot it loosely around your neck like a necklace. And you can use it while nursing or to shade the baby later as well. If you want to.

- The most comfortable and supportive bra you can afford. Have a proper fitting when you start growing out of it. Don't even think about nursing bras until around the eighth month.

- Comfortable shoes that are easy to put on, with arch support for preference. Pregnancy changes your centre of gravity and this affects your weight distribution. Additionally, your feet will almost definitely swell (which can be uncomfortable) and you may go up a shoe size. Consider practical sneaker style loafers for everyday errands, flip flop sandals for when you can't get shoes on and a pretty pair of flats for going out.

General purchasing notes:

- Buy clothes when you need them, with just the next few months in mind - both leading up to and after childbirth. You don't know how

Signature Wardrobe Planning

your body is going to change and the same concerns about budget wastage apply.

- Look for stretchy microfibres.

- Look for A-line, empire line, or wrap tops and dresses as these are more likely to accommodate your expanding breasts and belly.

- Side ruching will give your belly room to expand into the fabric excess, and compress back to disguise post baby belly making the garment wearable for longer.

- Thick straps and sleeves will hide bra straps and manage the changes in bust size.

- Button front shirts can be worn tied and as jackets.

- Consider other clothes that can do double duty for nursing as well.

Age

I hesitated to include this in the list because I don't think your age should affect your decisions about what you wear any more than your body size, shape or skin colour does (and I know they all do). If it fits, makes you happy, is appropriate for the activities you are doing in the places you are doing them, then it is appropriate for You.

Not everyone feels this way. Some people think that "old" people should routinely wear more concealing clothes, though no one is really game to tell you at what age you must lay aside your youthful clothes. The truth is that there are some older people who are physically in better shape than some younger ones, and there are some younger people who prefer to dress more modestly than some older ones. There are no rules.

Advice from 1925 suggests that older people should be taking leadership, and demonstrating the principles of dressing beautifully and appropriately in a dignified way. You should be keeping physically and mentally fit so that you can dress well for as long as you can. And while you shouldn't follow fashion as slavishly as you once did, you should adapt it to your shape and colouring. Your clothes should be the highest quality possible, in rich, good quality fabrics, neatly made in the right colours and shapes. They should be easy to get in and out of with convenient closures. Perhaps the very elderly may be permitted lose soft clothing, in colours, lines and fabrics to enhance and conceal as best for them.

From a practical perspective, you may want to consider the impact of things like arthritis, vision loss and balance deterioration on your ability to dress yourself.

Faintheartedness

Similarly, you might constrain yourself through concern about what friends and family might think. You might buy clothes for a life you don't live and events you will never go to because that's what *they* think is suitable. These clothes won't make you happy - how could they when they are not appropriate for you?

I don't think you need to worry too much about serious repercussions to your clothing choices. You are unlikely to face the terror and danger of events like the 1920s New York Hat Riots, where men were beaten up and had their straw boaters smashed for wearing them past September 15 (the unofficial day for reverting to felt winter hats).

Some people think that caring about what you wear and how you look is wrong. They might call it vanity, egotistical, or perhaps narcissistic. It's an interesting modern interpretation. In 1925, women were advised to take a "wholesome pride" in their personal grooming and dressing well; increasing not only their own happiness but that of those around them. And by 1937 it had become your *duty* to dress well, not just for your sake, but for the sake of those who had to look at you!

You should buy clothes that excite you, whether they are basics or staples or essentials or classics or neutrals or stars or statements or whatever you want to call them. And you should wear them. There is no reason why you shouldn't choose your everyday shirt with as much love, care and attention as your Christmas dinner dress. In fact, it deserves even more love and attention because you will wear it more often.

If you always buy clothes that you love and are appropriate for your lifestyle, you will never have to worry about being improperly dressed. You can confidently put your best foot forward, make the best of any situation and be your authentic charming self, because you *know* that you look good.

SUMMARY

Once you have determined your budget, you need to think about your:

- willingness to take care of your clothes
- climate
- region
- career
- leisure activities
- age
- faintheartedness

so that you can build your wardrobe with clothes that are appropriate for the life you lead.

CHAPTER 9

Step 3: Establish Your Style

Style, similar to appropriateness, is all about YOU. It is your distinctive presentation of your authentic self. It has a component of grooming, behaviour and deportment (the way that you move and speak). It does not specifically mean elegant or fashionable. It is not a fixed thing, it is fluid because your knowledge and tastes are always changing.

In 1925, you were advised that you had the right to be beautiful, but that to do this you needed to eat well, exercise and take fresh air to encourage a good complexion and healthy hair. You could further enhance your general appearance with a little makeup and the right hairstyle. Your individual expression of your beauty was considered an asset. Oddly, this is the thing that most modern women have a lot of trouble with.

It's worth pointing out that if you don't make the effort to define your style, someone else will define it for you. Which is probably why modern women have a lot of trouble understanding they are beautiful.

Not to mention that the period in which you are young and beautiful enough to be thoughtlessly fashionable is so much shorter than the rest of your life. The sooner that you can define your style, the more heartache you will save yourself when you find you have passed your fashion use by date.

WHAT IS STYLE ANYWAY?

Style blends your opinions about what is beautiful with what is appropriate. It's not just what you wear, but how you wear it too - your posture and carriage. You improve fashion by using it to express yourself; *choosing* to dress well gives you style and influence.

You already know this is not something you are born with (unless you are very lucky). You have to learn it; perhaps you have been lucky enough to have a good teacher, but it's more likely you haven't had anyone to guide you through this.

The foundation of *your* style is your pride in yourself and your appearance. It's wearing correctly fitting underwear that supports your posture and lies neatly under your clothes. It's walking lightly and gracefully, perhaps carrying something to keep your hands busy, while you stand comfortably and neatly in a manner that is in keeping with your clothing.

Discovering your style requires effort. You need to analyse what others are wearing, training your eye to understand how the lines, accessories and appropriateness of stylish clothes differ from mediocre ones.

BODY SHAPE

Expressing your style began as a way to emphasise your "good" points and suppress your "bad". Of course to do this you have to spend some time in front of the mirror being quite honest with yourself.

Signature Wardrobe Planning

I used to find it quite hard to see the whole of me in the mirror rather than focussing on what I thought of as my chunky calves or flabby belly. I changed my perspective by trying on a lot of different clothes in stores and taking photos of them. Then I printed them (several to a page) and looked at them as if they were a magazine spread, and I was quite surprised to find that among other things, my calves weren't that chunky nor my belly that flabby. I think this is a valuable exercise you really should consider, because other people do not look at you the same way that you look at yourself.

Moving forward, I use a full-length mirror in a very ornate frame. I find it helps me to stand back from it and look at myself as if I am a painting hanging in an art gallery; it's easier to see and critique a painting's lines and colours than your own body. And when you think about it, this is *exactly* how your friends see you when they stand on the street waiting for you to catch up with them.

Understanding your body shape helps you to dress it well, and "correct" irregularities, for example, not shortening yourself more if you are petite or stretching yourself if you are tall.

At this point, you may be expecting a long list of things to correct and advice on how to do that, but not in this book! That's because you are a unique individual, the sum of your parts, not a bunch of problems that require correction. If I was going to concede that there are problems to be corrected, it is the clothes that need correcting not you. And by the way, almost all of that correcting advice is contradictory.

For example, at 4' 11", I am too short for "petite" clothes... "Conventional" wisdom suggests that I should wear tiny skirts, tiny patterns and tiny pieces of jewellery. Or as I think of it, dolls clothes. But actually, I want people to treat me like a grown up and dressing like a doll is not going to achieve that. And even worse, as a short leg owner, I should wear skirts that end just below the knee and as a chunky calve owner I should not wear skirts that end just below the knee. My short neck apparently requires low necklines, but my full bust forbids them. My short waist forbids waist cinching yet my full middle requires it. I'm sure you understand the problem.

However, if you understand your body's proportions, regardless of whether the fashion is for dropped waists, short skirts or big shoulders you will be able to ensure that yours are the right size for you. These proportions apply equally to all different body sizes and shapes, and that's because they are based on the Ancient Greek science of Geometry (you were wrong when you said you would never use math when you grew up).

The Greeks used geometric principles when they designed those beautiful statues we admire so much. They identified that irregular spacing looks more attractive than regular spacing, did some complicated calculations and figured out that halfway between a third and a half makes a strangely interesting division that is more attractive than the others. Regardless of the size of the thing you are portioning - your body, your dress or your skirt.

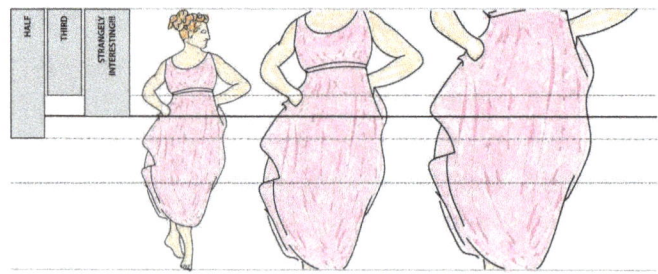

Figure 1: The Greek Law of Space Division

And you can divide the proportions infinitely (if you want).

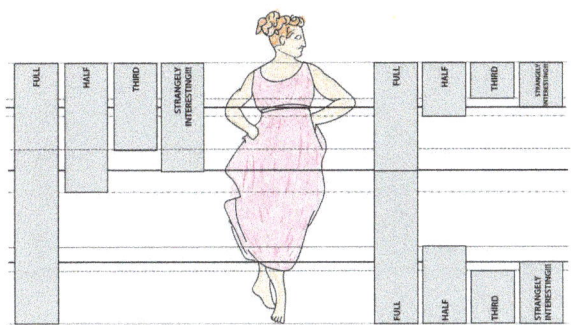

Figure 2: More Strangely Interesting Divisions

And this comes in handy when you put together an outfit for working out nice proportions.

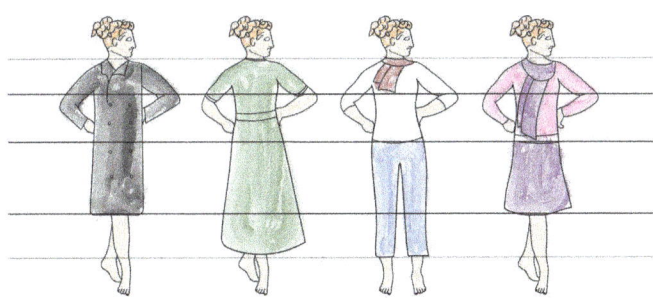

Figure 3: Outfit Divisions

Some say you can use this to change your apparent size and shape - vertical or horizontal stripes, big or small patterns. But as with the other figure correction advice, there are as many pattern variations as there are people so just try the clothes on, take a picture and see what you think. You might like it.

Similarly, knowing how proportions work for you is useful for bringing cohesion to your overall look, by ensuring that accessories are correctly placed.

The easiest way for you to work this out is more or less what I have done here. Take a photo of yourself and measure your height. Then calculate your half, thirds and strangely interesting dimensions. Print your photo and draw lines where your measurements are, similar to Figure 2. These lines can help you decide where your necklaces, waists and hems should be, but remember that these dimensions can be for individual items of clothing as well as your body.

Colour Selection

With your body proportioned, you can move onto colour selection, and this relies on some knowledge of colour theory. It's important to get this right because colour enhances or detracts from a garment's fabric and line (as well as your skin and hair). I'm sure you've had the experience of buying the same thing in two or more colours but finding you prefer one over the other(s).

You could take the easy way out and use a personalised colour service that will categorise you into a season and give you examples of approved colours. However, exact colours will not always be available and if you don't understand what makes them your colours you may not be able to confidently substitute.

The colour spectrum is a continuum, not the seven distinct colours we see in the rainbow (red, orange, yellow, green, blue, indigo, violet). In between each of these colours are others generally labelled by those that make them up, for example, blue-green. It is actually a circle joined at the red and violet ends to form what we know as the colour wheel.

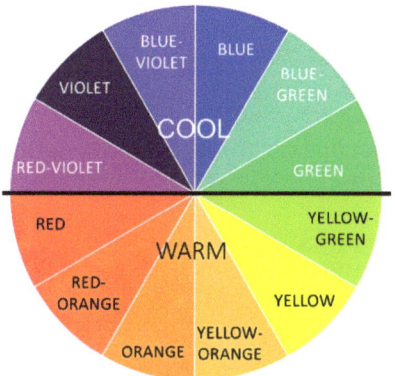

Figure 4: The Colour Wheel

The primary colours red, yellow and blue combine to create secondary colours orange, green and violet. Mixing secondary produces the tertiaries citrine, olive and russet. Mixing tertiary forms colour greys (as opposed to natural grey which is a blend of black and white), which don't have names because they are hard to reproduce.

Colours have characteristics.

- Hues are the colours that result when a little of one is added to another.

- Values are variations of light (added white) and dark (added black). Tints are light values and the shades dark values.

- Intensity refers to the purity of the colour, saturated colours are full intensity and natural grey the least pure.

- Warm colours are mainly reds and yellows.

- Cool colours mostly blues and green.

- Retiring colours are inconspicuous, generally very dark and lacking in warmth, such as seal grey, bottle green or greyed tan.

- Pastels are the lightest colours.

Colour schemes can be:

- Monochromatic (different values and intensities of one colour).

- Analogous (a combination of adjacent colours e.g. blue and blue-violet).

- Complementary (contrasting - opposites on the colour wheel, e.g. yellow and violet).

- Neutral (contrasting neutrals e.g. white on black).

You can observe different colour schemes on show in nature, museums and art exhibitions, store windows and other people's clothes. Or look at the Adobe Colour website and muck about with themes to see what they look like here: https://colour.adobe.com/create/colour-wheel.

The reason this is important is that the colours you wear change the way your skin and hair are perceived. I'm sure you've had the experience of people asking whether you are ill when you feel fine.

This is also why you shouldn't believe you can't wear orange (for example) it's just a matter of finding the correctly hued and tinted orange for you.

And why it's *really* important to separate your coloured clothes in the wash.

Unfortunately, colours also change under different lighting conditions, which is one reason why you have been disappointed when you got your new clothes home and tried them on with your existing wardrobe. Where possible try clothes on in light close to the lighting you will be wearing them in. And try them on with the accessories you intend to wear with them.

Colours also have the effect of expressing your personality. People who wear dark colours are generally expected to be sober and reserved and those who wear brighter colours are expected to be more outgoing which can be surprising for the people you are with if you get it wrong. Understanding your colours also helps you choose the new fashion ones that will work for you.

One suggestion from 1925 is to dress for your eyes during the day and your hair at night. For example, delft blue will look crisp during the day and unremarkable at night, whereas scarlet may be too striking for daytime but enhance dark hair at night. Of course, if you are a striking woman, you may be comfortable wearing red during the day, so by all means do.

The best colour choices enhance your skin and hair as well as your eyes. You can often identify them by looking at old photos of yourself (or making another magazine spread), but you might prefer to have a colour consultation or buy an app to help. Your natural colouration may change over time, and this can be managed with makeup. However, it is better to work at making sure the correct hues, tints and tones are purchased in your main clothes, their trimmings and your accessories. The wrong hair colour can also skew results.

Commonly the wardrobe building advice was to pick a colour palette and stick with it; a dark base colour supplemented by one or two harmonising colours in your accessories. You might prefer dark for winter, with a lighter shade for summer. If you find that you need to start from the beginning, this is a good approach to take to ensure you get the best value.

Personality

Your clothing shapes and colours combine with your personality to convey who you are. And there cannot be any compromise here, because compromising is not being true to yourself, and this deceives others.

In 1925, the Woman's Institute of Domestic Arts and Sciences used four personality types:

1. **Youthful:** a person that retains their youthful outlook and manner their whole life and consequently chooses simple clothing in bright colours, busy patterns and fluffy designs.

2. **Feminine:** soft flowing fabrics, pastel shades in loose full styles.

3. **Dignified:** draped clothes in dark subdued colours, and richly textured fabrics.

4. **Tailored:** actively participates in business and sport, and may appear to have severely tailored features. They are best in plain clothes made from stiff fabrics with severe lines.

A more recent version of this gives us:

1. **Sporty Natural:** the "girl next door" easy going and comfort driven dresser.

2. **Feminine Romantic:** has a delicate soft appearance and prefers soft colours, flowing silhouettes.

3. **Tailored Classic:** understated and elegant, prefers balance and symmetry.

4. **High-Fashion Dramatic:** the clotheshorse who prefers a striking, head-turning look.

Other descriptions I have seen include:

Signature Wardrobe Planning

- Eclectic, Bohemian, Maverick and Bombshell
- Creative, Romantic, Casual and Elegant
- Expressive, Ladylike, Relaxed, Dramatic

These are the same basic personalities (listed in the same order), just described a little differently in a way that reflects societal change. If I had the space to wax lyrical about each of these personalities you would see aspects of yourself in each of them. I'd say I'm about 59% tailored (4), 22% youthful (1), 16% feminine (2) and 3% dignified (3). No one is 100% one personality type, but each of us has a default we use when we are not pretending to be someone else.

For the sake of consistency, I am going to refer to them as types one through four for the rest of this book.

As the fourth personality, my natural lean is towards structured garments in pure saturated hues. You might prefer bright patterned flounces (one), or soft pastel coloured clothing (two), or chunky knits in rich autumnal colours (three).

Your personality also guides you in the little details, do you prefer:

- pockets that you can shove things into or do you the smooth unbroken line that comes without pockets?
- small compact bags or big ones with studs and tassels and zips (and so on)?
- 5" stilettos or 2" Cuban heels?
- genuine animal skins or manufactured ones?

All these tiny individual choices made over and again each shopping trip can be rolled into your general purchasing principles so that you don't have to think about them all the time.

You might think this makes it difficult for each personality to find something appropriate to wear for all the activities they undertake, from business to sport to eveningwear. But having an idea of your fashion personality actually makes it easier for you to identify the colours and styles you need. For example, in cardigans the first personality type might prefer cute and brightly patterned, the second a soft, shapeless grey, the third woman a thick textured burgundy, and the fourth smooth and closely fitted black. Knowing which personality type you are makes it easy to bypass all the other styles.

Just like colours, there are many services that you can use to type yourself, again usually into one of four types. There are also services that will translate your Myers-Briggs (and the like) results into a system for getting dressed.

Confidence

As I mentioned in step two, sometimes you buy clothes from faintheartedness, rather than from confidence. If you have been pretending to be someone else, it will be hard to turn aside from that and learn to trust and appreciate your judgement when it comes to the clothes you wear.

I also mentioned the need to examine yourself dispassionately and learn to see your body as a whole, not just a collection of body parts you don't like. Taking a constant stream of photos helps you see why some shapes, colours, fabrics and patterns work for you and others don't. But if you don't look, you won't ever see.

The easiest way to develop your confidence is to start with a small group of looks that you know work for you. I started with one outfit: plain black jeans and a long sleeved semifitted red tunic. Over time, I expanded that to include a navy and white striped Breton t-shirt, a loose short sleeved red and blue floral top (which I had to shorten and shape after a few wears). Now and again I add something new, like a navy A-line skirt with one big red and white flower, and then a red cardigan to go with the skirt and the floral top.

I've made mistakes, like a linen Liberty floral print button up shirt… I now understand that neither the fabric nor the pattern was compatible with the formality of the shirt's structure. And I remembered I just don't like tiny prints (dolls clothes).

These sorts of small hard-won kernels of knowledge help you understand who you are and what your style is. And this understanding gives you the confidence to dress in a way that is authentically and appropriately you.

Signatures

You might be wondering when I was getting to signatures. Most people think of Steve Job's black turtlenecks, or Anna Wintour's dresses when it comes to signatures, but I don't want to put you in the same outfit every day. Even assuming you wanted to wear the same thing every day.

Your signature look is an outward manifestation of who you are, not an indicator that you can't put an outfit together. If all your purchases take into account what is appropriate and stylish for you, you will begin to develop a look that is uniquely and identifiably you.

If you were so inclined, you might call it your personal brand. Perhaps it's because you almost always wear blue A-line skirts and never black pencil skirts, or that you love polka dots and loathe stripes, or have a collection of beautiful vintage silk scarves. The general purchasing principles you have been developing as you work through this book are bringing that look into existence.

To help with this, some people give themselves style keywords to guide their planning and shopping, kind of like interior design terms like "shabby chic" that give you an instant picture of what the look is all about. Some that I have heard include "nouvelle chic", "modern mod", "glamour grunge", "elegant bohemian" and "modest retro". They don't make sense to me, but they're not my words so why would they? (For the record, mine are "opulently chic" – I'm a work in progress).

You could also create a mood board by collecting pictures of outfits you love (in a notebook or on Pinterest), noting what you like about the outfit and how you think it will fit with your life. I love the kind of big skirted girly dresses my mother put me in when I was a child, but they are not appropriate for my life right now. However, I could take inspiration from them by including large-scale patterns, roses and fit and flare dresses into my wardrobe.

The Exception that Proves the Rule

There are times in life when you need to change your look and/or level up, like when you leave college and start work, you or your partner are promoted, you marry a millionaire or have kids. These are just some of the possible real life aspirational and transitional scenarios. At these times, your authentic self is in transition between one kind of normal and another, and it can be difficult to know where to start adjusting your wardrobe.

The first thing to do is to remember that you are still you. All those little decisions about pockets, skirt shapes and colours are all still your guiding purchasing principles. You just need to work out how to translate them for your new life.

The easiest way to do that is to find a fashion inspiration or mentor to copy, and I recommend a real person, not a television or movie character, nor a celebrity as their costumes will probably be too highly sexualised. You can also start developing a mood board as described in the Signatures section. In chapter 17 (Decoding Dress Codes) I make some suggestions about Job Interview dress codes which might help with the work related scenarios. New wives of rich men, might be better to focus on luxurious high-quality fabrics.

It *will* feel strange and uncomfortable for a time, for example, transitioning from stretchy cardigans to firm jackets will take an enormous effort of will, but if you persevere you will become accustomed to your new normal.

Summary

Developing your own clothing style takes into account your:

- body shape,
- skin, hair and eye colour,
- personality type.

Clothes that accommodate these will give you the confidence that you are always dressed the right way for you.

CHAPTER 10

Step 4: Decide Your Needs

There is a lot of confusion over what clothes we *need* (as opposed to *want*). This is not helped by each new list of "essential" wardrobe items released by whatever clothing guru is on top of the pile at the moment. Most of the items on these lists are completely irrelevant to the life I lead, and maybe yours too. I'm fairly confident that no-one will ever *need* a pair of metal studded shoes (unless there *really* is a zombie apocalypse in which case I recommend very big studs).

At the very least, your clothing should fulfil three criteria;

1. preserve your health by keeping you warm and protecting you from injury,

2. allow unrestricted movement so that you can freely undertake the activities you need to,

3. be sufficiently "decent" (respectable or presentable) to permit participation in social and community events like dinners or the movies.

In 1918, an ideal wardrobe contained only nine items of clothing (four or five day dresses, an afternoon dress, evening dress, a blouse and a skirt). There was very little change over the next couple of decades; but by 1936 the nine items had become a coat, suit, two day dresses, afternoon dress, evening dress and ski suit (or overcoat).

Yet in 2005 one magazine recommended 36 items, and another recommended 40 in 2008. In 2007, yet another magazine recommended purchasing 20 items of clothing, six pairs of shoes plus accessories and hosiery valued at $18,000 for ONE month's wear.

Fortunately, after working through the last three steps (and jotting a few notes), you have all the information necessary to start working out how many clothes *you* need. It might be nine, or it could be 40, you are the only one that knows what you really need.

Just in case you are wondering what to do with all this information, we can start by examining what ordinary working families did in 1928. These particular families belonged to men building railway lines; some were itinerant workers living in camps beside the tracks, some lived in nearby towns:

- they put money aside for shoe repairs, laundry services saved for big purchases like coats.

- for the most part, they did not have running water, or in some cases electricity so it's likely that they would have worn one set of clothing while the other was in the 1900 six tub wash.

- their purchases show a definite seasonal focus, with a half summer half winter annual spend.

- they bought two sets of everyday (work/school) clothes, and two to three sets of underwear person per annum.

Signature Wardrobe Planning

- when money was tight, they prioritised father's work clothes (income provider), followed by the children and last of all mother.

- they bought one set of good clothes to wear to Church and the movies, giving priority to wife and children (to demonstrate respectability).

Obviously you don't have a 1928 style life, but their spending is a viable starting template for your wardrobe planning:

- spend two-thirds on everyday/working clothes and one on good/leisure

- include provisions for winter and/or summer

- annual refresh of socks/stockings and underwear

- include savings towards irregular big purchases such as overcoats

- include dry cleaning and alteration costs

Reading between the lines of the survey results, there are also some hidden tips:

- don't buy clothes for places you don't go

- be patient; building a cohesive wardrobe takes time

- conservative dress looks stylish longer than following fads

- taking good care of your clothes maximises their useful lives

- revise your wardrobe plan periodically to incorporate changes in your body as well as fashion

This knowledge provides your framework, but there are still some other things to take into consideration.

Replacement Cycles

I have been tracking my purchases and disposals for a few years now, and because of this I know that:

- my jeans last two to three years
- a t-shirt one year
- hiking socks three years
- everyday underwear one year, fancy hand-washed underwear two years

I spoke with a tailor a few years ago (I wanted to have a suit made and we were chatting), and he said that a well-made and cared for wool overcoat could last for 15 years, and a well-made and cared for wool suit worn every day with bottoms dry cleaned fortnightly would last five to ten. Of course, cheaper clothes that are badly made in lower quality fabrics, and not cared for will not last as long.

Favourite Cycles

Favourites relates a little to laundry cycles. I'm not sure if you have heard of the Pareto principle? Also known as the 80/20 rule. Basically, it explains that 20% of the effort brings 80% of the reward. Or in wardrobe terms that you wear 20% of your clothes 80% of the time. Or round about that, but you know that you wear some of your clothes a lot, and some not much at all. This is partly the reason why you feel drawn to multiples of some items. Working out what your 20% is can help you stop buying the 80% (which is what your purchasing principles are for).

Fashion Cycles

Fashion cycles are related to both replacement and favourite cycles as well - you might be wearing something long past its use by date. Maybe you don't want to let go of the good times, or you haven't noticed that time has left you behind.

Regardless of that, when the time comes to replace it you will not be able to find an exact copy. But you can analyse what you like about it (e.g. the shape, the length, the colour) and use that information to buy something similar. Or perhaps take it to a dressmaker as a pattern for a modern remake.

It also relates back to accessories and colours. Accessories are generally less expensive than your other clothes, and no one will notice that you are wearing the same basic outfit if you are wearing a striking scarf, necklace, earrings or the like as well. Except maybe your mother.

How to Build an Outfit

Within those limitations, one of the main problems you will have building your wardrobe is starting where you are. Almost all the advice suggests or implies that you need to throw everything out and start from scratch, but I don't think that's necessary. I think that you can (and should) start where you are. After all, you have favourites! Also, it might take you a little time to decide what moves from the maybe list to the buy list, and you will probably need something to wear in the meantime.

That's not to say that you can't get rid of things that you have already decided are not appropriate or stylish enough for you. But before you do, you might want to make some notes about why you don't think they are right for you anymore (take a look at chapters 12 [Record Keeping], 13 [How to Conduct a Wardrobe Review] and 14 [How to Create a Capsule

Wardrobe] for hints). This will help you avoid the same "mistakes" in the future.

So where to start? For this, we turn to 1935 when the wardrobe building advice was to collect together a small number of appropriate and stylish outfits. Their idea of appropriate dress was more formal than is customary today and their outfit consisted of a dress, supported by shoes, hosiery, handbag, jewellery, umbrella, hat, gloves, coat and the correct underwear. Naturally, the more of your dresses these supporting clothes go with, the better, and this is where the planning comes in.

Each of your outfits has its own theme or purpose (they called it "spirit" which sounds so much better), and it is expressed through shared colour, texture and/or consistency of line and detail. The theme draws against your personality and illustrates your relationships; for example, your entertaining at home eveningwear will represent freedom and enjoyment regardless of colours and materials, while your event eveningwear expresses leisure and camaraderie in exotic and fanciful fabrics and details. I'm going to assume that I don't need to tell you that these items need to fit well.

Other purpose examples include:

- dignified and attractive for Church.

- fashionable but not too dressy for bridge clubs, concerts and lectures.

- tailored and serviceable for shopping.

It works like this, your:

- outfit is based on your dress, which provides the colour and textural base.

Signature Wardrobe Planning

- shoes suit the scale of your body, and their colour intensity sustains and emphasises the overall harmony and balance of your outfit.

- hat and gloves match your outfit purpose (i.e. don't wear your gardening gear with your city dresses). Your hat should repeat the lines of your body and face, and your gloves should not be too distinctive (because you will be wearing them with a variety of outfits).

- hosiery is the right colour intensity, texture and design for your skin and/or outfit (e.g. semi-sheer mid weight with your tweed suit).

- handbag can make or break your outfit. It should harmonise with your hat, shoes and gloves. Additionally, it should complement the trimmings of your dress or match the overall tone of your outfit, and harmonise with the lines of your outfit.

- accessories such as jewellery should enhance the line and colour of, and add interest to your outfit. Ideally they will be in keeping with your personality and stage of life. The fall of the piece should repeat the lines of your body, shape of the face and length of the neck. If you still use handkerchiefs they should be plain white or match your outfit.

- underwear is really important - it protects you from the weather and skin irritations caused by your dress, and protects your dress from your perspiration and body oils. Their tightness, elasticity and comfort play an important role in determining the style of your dress. They should match your theme, e.g. plain and practical for street wear or sheer and dainty for the evening. Regardless they should be soft against the skin and easy to clean.

As I mentioned, we don't dress this formally anymore, but if you take a moment and imagine yourself in a dress, and then put on a skirt and a jacket, then a skirt and a top, and then pants and a top. You can now see that these things can all be the dress in the above outfit.

So let's go to the other extreme and imagine blue jeans and a green t-shirt for a day of running errands. Perhaps you will wear black leather ankle boots or green "dress" sneakers (as opposed to sports sneakers). Handbags are very personal things, and you probably already know which one you would use with this outfit, so I'm just going to suggest you keep it as plain (or elaborate) as your jeans, t-shirt and shoes, and at a scale that is in proportion to your body. And the same with your jewellery - maybe plain metallic hoop earrings or a simple chain with pendant. And plain comfortable undies. For your jacket or coat, you might choose a blue denim or black leather, or maybe a lightweight cardigan.

Your theme (and personality) is also useful for the practical details of your outfits. Say your errand outfit was a skirt and blouse. You might want pockets to put pens or tissues in, but you might prefer pockets concealed in the seams rather than patched on the hip or breast. You might *like* pussy bow blouses but because the ties aren't really practical for you, *choose* a round neckline and wear a bold necklace instead.

ONLY BUY WHAT YOU WILL USE

I think that somewhere along the line, we picked up on the importance of looking respectable when we left the house, but not what the most practical and sustainable way of doing that was. Assuming our mothers knew this. My own wardrobe problems have often been caused by too many Princess (good) Clothes and not enough Cinderella (everyday) ones, and when

Katy and I talked about this she said she was the same, so perhaps we all do this. Not that Princess Clothes are a bad thing, but there are Princess Clothes you will wear and Princess Clothes you probably won't ever have the opportunity to wear.

From that point of view, I think 1928 forms a good example - prioritise Cinderella, not the Princess. But you need to know what your particular Cinderella clothes are first - maybe a suit with five business shirts is appropriate for you, or maybe two pairs of jeans and five t-shirts. And your version of good clothes might be crystal studded dark wash jeans or perhaps the archetypal little black dress you can dress up or down.

At this point you should have a good idea of the clothing forms and styles of clothes that you need, but before you go ahead and buy anything it's a good idea to conduct a wardrobe review to see what you already have and use (see chapter 13).

Summary

The clothes that you need depend on what's appropriate for you, and what you think is stylish. Allocate your overall purchases according to how you will use them:

- spend two-thirds on everyday clothes (career, leisure) and one on good.
- provisions for winter and/or summer.
- annual refresh socks/stockings, underwear.
- savings towards irregular big purchases such as overcoats.
- dry cleaning and alteration costs.

Take into account

- replacement cycles

- favourite cycles
- fashion cycles

Remember that the key to pulling an outfit together this way is choosing:

- colours that harmonise with your skin.
- similar textures, e.g. boucle with chunky beads, not fine chains.
- consistent details, e.g. a plain, structured work dress with a plain utilitarian collar (not fancy lace).

CHAPTER 11

Modern Day Worked Example

I don't know about you, but I *really* dislike books that tell you here's the information, work it out for yourself. So I'm including two examples at opposite ends of the Womenswear spectrum to show you how the same basic information applies in different contexts.

This is actually a wild stab at what these women might require; I was an Emily a few years back but I have never been an Amanda. I took Amanda's prices from Macy's and Emily from J Crew and Nordstrom, but I imagine if you are one of them you have a much better idea of where you would go.

STEP 1: SET YOUR BUDGET

I've given them both the same example income of $50,000 per annum, which after tax leaves $42,203. Their 15% clothing budget is $6,330.

- "Amanda" is married with children, and has a 30% share of the budget which is $1,899. A 2:1 split gives her $1,272 for everyday wear and $627 for good.

- "Emily" is unmarried (no children) which means that the entire $6,330 is hers to spend; $4,241 for everyday and $2,089 for good.

STEP 2: DETERMINE YOUR APPROPRIATE

Clothing Care

- Amanda feels like she is always washing clothes and doesn't want to have to make a special effort on her own right now. She would prefer not to hand wash or iron.

- Emily is too busy having fun to spend a lot of time caring for her clothes. She prefers to send them to a cleaner.

Climate

- With warm summers but cold winters, Amanda needs warm layers for winter.

- Emily has hot summers and cool winters and could possibly manage with just an extra layer.

Region

- Amanda lives in a small town, and needs a car to get around, but she doesn't need any special clothing to manage this.

- Emily lives in a big city, mostly walks and catches public transport. She just needs "walking" shoes and a lightweight overcoat.

Career

- Amanda is a stay at home Mum who keeps house, grows vegetables and ferries her kids around. She needs practical and durable clothes that don't require special care.

- Emily works in an air-conditioned office where formal presentation (suit) is required. She would like to attract more respect from her colleagues.

Leisure Activities

- Amanda mainly attends Church and church-related activities, kids sporting activities, wider family dinners and parties. She meets other mums for coffee, and goes on date nights with her husband. She doesn't need formal clothes because her everyday clothes are suitable for most of her activities. She wants nice clothes for church, but not so nice they can't be worn for other activities.

- Emily eats out with friends and goes on dates, as well as visiting galleries, museums and concerts. She needs some formal wear for work events, semi-formal for gallery openings and so on, and smart casual for lunches, shopping and the like.

Health

- Amanda has good general health. She occasionally needs elbow strapping for garden work but doesn't require specialised clothing for this.

- Emily really feels the cold and needs some kind of layer to hand at work, and often a light cover up in summer.

Age

- Amanda doesn't feel age is relevant, but would like to dress like a more mature woman.

- Emily doesn't think age is an issue but feels a need to look fashionable.

Faintheartedness

- Amanda is concerned about what her husband, parents and church might think, and she doesn't want to appear vain.

- Emily is afraid of looking out of date (and touch) and worries that it makes her appear as though she isn't capable at work.

STEP 3: ESTABLISH YOUR STYLE

Body Shape

- Amanda thinks she's too fat, would like to drop a few pounds, and wants to hide her thighs and tummy.

- Emily is fairly happy with her overall shape though admits she doesn't fit the current fashion requirement for skinniness. She would like some muscle definition and is thinking about joining a gym.

Colour Selection

- Amanda is tired of dark practical colours and wants some girly dusky pinks and purples.

- Emily has a lot of black (it is the City after all), but wears reds and blues, is thinking about bringing in some yellow for contrast.

Personality

- Amanda resonates with personality type two (Feminine/Romantic). She likes loosely draped clothing in soft textures. She thinks she is living the feminine dream, but didn't realise happy ever after would be so messy.

- Emily is personality type four (Tailored/High-Fashion Dramatic) and while she wouldn't call herself high fashion dramatic, she doesn't want to look like everyone else. She prefers fitted coloured clothing and this does make her stand out.

Confidence

- Amanda lives in jeans, and t-shirts but would prefer to dress up a little more.

- Emily loves a knee length skirt or dress with a long fitted jacket.

STEP 4: DECIDE YOUR NEEDS

These thoughts help to put your basic shopping list together.

Table 4: Draft Shopping List

"Amanda"		"Emily"	
Everyday Staples			
3 sets underwear	$150	4 sets underwear	$500
sports bra	$50	10 pairs tights	$100
3 socks	$20		$600
long johns & camisole	$100		
	$320		

Draft Shopping List Cont.

"Amanda"		"Emily"	
Everyday Career			
jeans	$175	skirt suit	$400
5 t-shirts	$100	matching pants	$150
cardigan	$50	matching dress	$200
sneakers	$50	4 blouses	$400
sandals	$50	cashmere cardigan	$350
	$425	wrap	$100
		pumps	$250
			$2,300
Everyday Leisure			
dress	$150	jeans	$300
skirt	$60	2 dresses	$500
2 blouses	$100	skirt	$150
	$310	3 blouses	$375
			$1,325
Good			
dress	$210	evening gown	$500
wrap	$80	2 cocktail dresses	$500
evening pumps	$100	evening wrap	$200
evening clutch	$75	evening pumps	$200
necklace	$100	evening clutch	$200
	$565	necklace	$300
			$1,900
Total Planned Expenditure			
$1,620		$6,125	
Available for Unplanned			
$279		$205	

Signature Wardrobe Planning

My lists for Amanda and Emily assume that they already have sufficient clothes and accessories, are replacing worn out clothes, and upgrading where they can. They both made some notes about changes of colour, so their replacement cycles will focus on incorporating those colours.

As discussed in Step One (Set Your Budget), you can save money by buying the things you know you want on sale. Amanda, has $150 pencilled in for three sets of underwear, but now that she has a wardrobe plan she has options:

- buy three sets on sale for $75 and put the difference towards something else
- buy three sets of higher priced on sale at $150
- buy six sets on sale for $150 and get rid of all her manky old ones
- buy three sets on sale, plus an additional three pairs of panties for $100
- decide her existing underwear is fine, buy one new set and put the balance towards something else

The final shopping list should be very detailed. For example, Amanda's "good" outfit should read more like this:

- pastel pink or coral chiffon ruched sleeveless dress ($210)
- gold tissue wrap ($80)
- gold evening pumps ($100)
- gold beaded clutch ($75)
- gold heart pendant necklace ($100)

Her list should have been drawn up taking into account the items she already owns (e.g. she has black patent Mary Janes that could work with the right accessories). She said she doesn't need a formal outfit, but that she wants nice clothes to wear to church and use for her other activities. She might be a little out of control in the Princess Clothes department here, but it could be that she is hoping her husband will take her somewhere very nice for their upcoming big number anniversary dinner. Or that she built the outfit from having fallen in love with the dress on a previous shopping expedition.

Having said that, with this level of detail, she can go straight for the pinks when she hits the store. And if she can't find a ruched sleeveless dress, she can tell by looking at her list that it won't matter a great deal if she buys the same style in a different colour. Or if she prefers the look and feel of a different pink dress that is $250 she has the information she needs to *decide* whether she buys that instead. She left herself $62 leeway for her good clothes so she could make that purchase as long as her other purchases remain close to budget.

Emily is thinking of joining a gym but hasn't made any provision for active wear. While it might be wise not to spend a lot of money until she knows she will use it, she could just as easily not join a gym because she doesn't have anything nice to wear when she goes.

Neither of our women has mentioned age as an issue, but Amanda wants to look more like a parent, and Emily wants more respect at work. Both of these can be addressed by working out what the issue is with their appearance. For example, Amanda predominantly wears jeans and t-shirts, and potentially looks more like the babysitter. If she can learn to comfortably dress differently, for example, in more structured blouses, she can make that leap.

Emily should look at more senior women in her office, identify how their dress and behaviour differs from hers, and start to copy the one(s) that most accurately represent where she wants to be.

Your final shopping list is not set in stone because life has a way of changing while you are not looking. Emily might be looking for a different job and decide to postpone her career purchases until she finds something. Her new job might be in a less formal workplace, so she might prefer patterned skirts and/or dresses that will go with her existing suit jackets instead. Or she might take a promotion in her current workplace and use her salary increase to invest in higher quality suiting.

It's also worth noting that it's a good idea not to commit your whole budget to purchases - I mentioned earlier that you should leave yourself space to save for future purchases. Emily's overcoat is five years old and while it still has plenty of life left in it, she wants cashmere next time so she's going to need to save $5,000 - $6,000 over the next few years.

Another good reason for leaving yourself a little space is that sometimes you see things that are just so wonderful you just can't imagine how life could possibly go on without them. A leopard print rain coat, Hawaiian print sneakers, vintage bakelite bangles - you name it there is something wonderful out there for everyone.

PART THREE:
Build and Maintain Your Wardrobe

HAVING WORKED THROUGH PART TWO, you now have an annual wardrobe plan. It is a living document that will grow and change as you and your circumstances do. This part helps you to extend it for three, five or as many years as is appropriate for you by tracking your purchases, reviewing what you own and deciding your future wardrobe direction.

CHAPTER 12

Record Keeping

It will probably not surprise you that I think good wardrobe planning requires an amount of record keeping. Calling it record-keeping sounds very grand, or perhaps too much like homework, but it's really just the notes you make as you write your wardrobe plan collected together into one place. You might prefer a notebook, an excel spreadsheet or an app - whatever works for you.

Keep as much or as little information as you need to make the purchasing decisions that are right for you. You may not want to be as detailed or specific as I am, and that's just fine.

The advice from 1949 is to work to a three-year plan, but you could choose a different schedule to work to depending on what your clothing needs are, for example, five yearly if you habitually wear suits, or two yearly if you wear mostly jeans. I work to a five-year plan, partly because I still think in terms of suits, and partly because I'm a natural planner. I would also like to ensure that I don't find myself too far behind the fashion eight ball by accident (by design is fine, but I'm sure we've all seen those women who never quite moved past their [1980s] glory days).

Clothing Records

First, you need to keep information about each garment you buy. This includes specifications (including brand, fabric, colour and size), your purchase and disposal dates and their total cost including alterations, postage and sale discounts.

As you do your six monthly wardrobe reviews (see the next chapter) categorise each as "go to", "favourite" and "mistake' according to what's appropriate and stylish for you. You might prefer other names like "best friends", "chocolate cake" or "chopped liver". You could colour them as well so you can see at a glance how you're doing with your purchases. Your colour ratios will get better over time, because as you come to understand what your mistakes are, you will make fewer and fewer of them.

This information also feeds through to your budget and replacement schedules. For example, I now know that I can expect my jeans to last two to three years because I bought my "go to" jeans in January 2012 (original price $175 + $10 to have the legs shortened) and disposed of them in March 2015.

In addition to purchasing information, you could maintain a separate inventory, updating it as you buy and dispose of items so that you always have a current list of what is in your wardrobe. If you are the kind of person who likes to plan their outfits ahead, you can try your new clothes on with your existing clothes, and track which items go with what. Or you could play Russian roulette to randomly pick an outfit.

Periodically review the clothing forms in your inventory to make sure you have a good balance. I like to be able to wear each garment with two or three others, so if I found that I was running low on tops I might need to prioritise those. Or perhaps more summer or winter clothes if I was short on them.

I used to keep track of how often I wore things but it didn't take long to become apparent that I am a 20% dresser. Tracking wears can be useful because it will help you see what you wear and if you make time to think about it, you will learn why you wear them. What, in particular, makes you put them on - the colour, the shape, the length, the trim, or the drape? And when you compare the number of wears to the total purchase price (including alterations and postage), you can calculate whether you think those purchases were good value.

You might also find that you wear particular clothing forms at particular times, for example, when you come home from the gym you always change into your fleecy sweats. Or that you never wear your fleecy sweats. This can help you understand the kinds of things that you don't like, for example, you have only been wearing your thick socks, and when you think about it, you realise that you have been standing a lot and your feet get sore so you prefer the extra padding.

Or you might find that you are buying clothes for a life you don't lead, for example, you may have changed jobs or left work and are still buying clothes to wear to your old workplace. This will give you an insight into what clothes you need, which will also feed into your replacement schedule.

Replacement Schedule

Your clothing records make it easy to start planning your shopping list, because they provide your replacement schedule.

For example, knowing that my jeans will last two to three years, tells me that if I want to maintain two pairs in rotation (one in the wash), on average I need to buy a new pair every year. Before I do anything else (on the assumption that I will always wear jeans) I know that they must go on my list for each of the years in my wardrobe plan. My house t-shirts last a year, my better quality street blouses two to three years. I don't replace my entire sock or underwear collection each year, but buy some pieces to top it up.

A friend who went into personal training told me that sneakers and sports bras used for fitness purposes should be replaced every six to twelve months depending on the fit and level of wear, so you can add them to your list too.

And if we go back to 1935 (when women had fewer items and wore them more often), everyday shoes would be replaced annually, dresses and blouses around two years, suits three to four years, and coats five to six years.

Now you have the start of your two, three or five-year wardrobe plan

Financial Records

These include your budget, expenditure and what's left. I divide the amount remaining by the number of months left in the year to give myself a monthly spend figure (so I don't go mad and spend it all at once) but you might prefer to link it to your paydays, or just track it annually. My budget includes alteration costs, makeup and jewellery, in the main because one year I went back and calculated that I had spent almost $500 on makeup, most of which I have never touched. (Ouch!)

Your clothing records also feed into your long-term budget preparation. For example, I use a five-yearly plan, and while I work on the current year the following five are pencilled in. It works this way:

- I know that I need to buy new jeans each year.
- I know the original purchase price was $185.

- I know that all other things being equal (though they never are), the same pair of jeans will cost more the second year (due to inflation, currency fluctuations and probably greed too).

- I add a margin of 5% to cover those costs, so (all other things being equal) the jeans will cost $185 + 5% = $194 in the second year.

- Then $194 + 5% = $204 in the third, $214 the fourth and $225 the fifth.

Not that clothing prices are so easily predictable. I will not be able to get exactly the same jeans again but it gives me a notional amount to pencil into my calculations. I can adjust this as the budget fleshes out. And if it turns out that I can buy jeans on sale for $150, then I can put the difference towards something else, or if more choose where to take it from.

Purchasing Principles

Having got this far, you have worked out what is appropriate and stylish for you, and you have developed purchasing principles to guide this year's shopping. Now you need to write them down in a short form to carry with you as a reminder.

These are the first purchasing principles I developed; yours will be different because your life is different to mine, but it will give you an idea about how you can express yours in a way that helps you plan out what you want to buy.

General Purchasing Principles:

1. simple classic styles
2. suitable for all occasions
3. suitable in both hot summers and cool winters
4. ideally everything matches everything else

5. made of natural fibres
6. best quality bra, shoes, bag, watch, glasses

Colour selections:

- **Main:** scarlet, royal blue, bright white
- **Neutral:** navy, black
- **Accent:** cerise
- **Accessories:** silver

Purchasing priorities:

- **Necessary:** street clothes and underwear
- **High:** to update look, comfortable shoes
- **Low:** hard to find items, nice to have, leisure and workout wear

My needs and purchasing principles have changed since then. For example, I probably don't need more than two levels of priorities (say necessary and fun). Katy has low, medium, high and a fourth super-urgent category for her signature crazy earrings. While there are some shapes of clothing I prefer (like flat front straight leg pants), as fashion changes so frequently it hasn't been practical for me to set limits on them. But having got this far, you might want to prescribe styles and colours, for example black knee length pencil skirts, loose coral calf length empire waist dresses or green fleecy cuffed sweat pants with patch pockets.

SHOPPING LIST

Your shopping list is basically your annual budget provisionally allocated by item. I call it a shopping list, but it's really

Signature Wardrobe Planning

more of a wish list; there will be some things that will be on it for years before you can find them. And some years you might buy more because some clothes are wearing quicker than expected or you might buy less because you have perfectly serviceable clothes in your closet that will do.

It is important to write everything you're planning down so when something unexpected comes up (like replacing your long johns because you accidentally left your old ones in your hotel and they haven't found them) you can make an informed decision about what to sacrifice to cover your purchase.

It should be very detailed; for example, that your summer dress should be a fitted white linen sundress with a flared skirt and your sandals should be white leather. These details are important for reminding you to stick to your list because you can immediately see that if you buy a black sun dress you need to rethink your sandals too

Many people conduct wardrobe reviews every six months (see chapter 13) at the changeover of the summer and winter seasons, and this can really help with wardrobe planning. If you find at the end of summer there really isn't much point putting your tattered swimsuit into storage, you can write it on your list when you discard it.

Your replacement schedule feeds into the list with annual replacements of things like jeans, hosiery and underwear that you can buy in the New Year sales. Theoretically these replacements are the most important things, but they are also the things that you have the most room for manoeuvre on in terms of cost and replacement frequency.

As you plan your purchases, note clothes that need alterations (e.g. my pant shortening at $10 per pair). When you complete your wardrobe reviews, you should also note any remodelling (e.g. shoes that need resoling, say $15) or repairs (resewing fallen hems, say $5) that are required and make provision for them on your list.

Examining again what is appropriate and stylish for you may add some new things into your list. For example, you might want to try a new colour in some accent pieces to see whether you can commit yourself. Or perhaps you realise you have been spending a lot of time over winter gardening and need some wellingtons for walking in the mud.

Other Records You Might Like the Idea Of

- An "Image Toolkit" containing pictures of your favourite outfits.

- Tags to hang on your clothes hangers telling you what each item goes with. Getting dressed might be a great trial if you forgot that it was red shirt day at work and you had discarded the skirt you usually wore your red shirt with.

- If you really care about being seen by the same people in the same outfit, a diary detailing what you wore, where and with whom can help with this. Or what you need to wear if you agree to meet someone in ten years' time at the top of the Empire State Building.

- A weekly planner so you can plan out what you're going to wear. Like menu planning for clothes - this one probably works best for those juggling different jobs or responsibilities with different levels of messiness.

- Records of your favourite brands, the places to get the best prices, the time of year, the name of your contact at the store and the like.

- Your appropriate lifestyle categories (e.g. career, sport, church) and your proportions of expenditure for each of them.

Signature Wardrobe Planning

- A mood board of looks, outfits, colours and styles that you like.

- Contact details for your favourite boutiques, dressmakers, and other relevant services.

- Somewhere to keep your store coupons and discount offers.

Summary

Tracking garment life cycles and full costs will provide the information you need for budgeting, determining what is appropriate for you and redefining you style.

CHAPTER 13

How to Conduct a Wardrobe Review

You probably cannot afford to buy a whole new wardrobe every season, and like most of us have to start with what you have. Some people prefer to review their wardrobes and then write their wardrobe plan, but I recommend doing it the other way around.

Your life moves ever forward, and your clothing requirements change though you might not always be aware of it. Things like you:

- are aiming for or have achieved a promotion at work and need to upgrade your appearance.

- now work from home and don't need the same level of formal work clothes.

- have become a stay at home carer of young, old or disabled people.

- have been diagnosed with a disease or condition and are under a new treatment regime.

Each of these, and many other life changes require a wardrobe rework, so I think it's worth rethinking what is appropriate and stylish for you at least annually. It's a waste of your budget to buy clothes that aren't going to work for you anymore (trust me, I've been there).

And it's worth remembering that building a wardrobe takes time, money and taste, and it needs to include renewal cycles that take account of changes in your skin, hair and body as well as fashion.

Review Cycle

The traditional haute couture calendar consists of two seasons; January - June and July - December. They were described as Spring (now called Spring/Summer or S/S for short) and Autumn (Autumn/Winter or A/W). It seems a handy way to break up your shopping, but in modern times not necessarily so easy:

- if you work in a nice climate controlled office you probably dress more or less the same all year round.

- if you live in the southern hemisphere and love particular northern hemisphere designers, you may be forced to buy your Autumn clothing in Spring (and vice versa).

- some stores and brands now offer mid-season collections such as "High Summer" or short-term collections such as "Resort Wear".

Nonetheless bi-annual wardrobe reviews are recommended by all sorts of people, and for those living in more extreme climates than me, the summer/winter wardrobe swap is the ideal time to do it.

Signature Wardrobe Planning

The actual weather conditions start to change at solstice/equinox dates (which change from year to year), so if you pick a date around about the 20th of March and September you'll be in the vicinity of spring/fall (autumn). Your own experience of your climate will guide you to the best time to swap over for you.

1. GET READY

This could be a difficult experience for you, and therefore everyone around you. Start by preparing yourself and making sure that your family/roommates go out for the day. Get yourself a glass of wine (not too much wine), cup of hot chocolate or other kind of treat, turn some of your favourite music up loud and get ready to go.

Gather some bags or boxes to categorise your clothes as you go. Potential labels include keep, trash, donate, sell, swap party, consign, tailor (alter), dry clean, kids dress up, store for the season, donate and so on. Pick which ones are relevant for you, and you could call them something inspirational like "soul-stirring" or similar that makes sense for you and hopefully makes the process more enjoyable.

Grab your wardrobe planning notebook and pen as you will be making notes about your clothes as you go. Also, if you live in a country that considers clothing donations to charities a tax deduction, you'll need to make some records.

2. GATHER ALL YOUR CLOTHES TOGETHER

Collect *every* single piece of clothing, shoe and accessory (including those in seasonal storage and waiting to be washed) and bring them to one place. Ideally somewhere clean. Perhaps your bed.

This will look horrendous, and you might want to do it a bit at a time, but it's important for you to *really* see what you have. You need to be able to compare the size of your various disposal piles to your keep piles to get a realistic idea of the adequacy of your previous shopping.

As you look at the pile of clothes, you might be able to just pull things out that you don't want anymore, identify clothes you thought you had lost or notice that you have multiples of things that at first glance don't seem too different. You might notice that you have a lot of blue and become aware that it makes you feel sad. Or see a sea of black and wonder where the colour is. Make a note of anything that seems important or that you want to think about later.

You will also have a gut feeling about which things are your "favourite", "go to" and "mistakes" and you should make a note of this for your future wardrobe planning. If you can identify why these items are in these groups you will be halfway to improving your next shopping trip almost immediately.

Just throw out all your tights, socks and underwear that are old, discoloured, stretched, worn, torn, holed, frayed and would generally embarrass you should the paramedics see them. Make a note in your book to replace them.

Thoroughly inspect each garment to ensure it is in good wearable condition; not stained, fraying or torn, has all its buttons, the zipper still works well, and so on. If you cannot mend or clean it, and aren't prepared to pay someone to do it, throw it in the trash.

Otherwise, try it on.

3. Try Everything On

Your goal for this step is to make sure that each garment in your closet still has a place in your life. Before you try on each

Signature Wardrobe Planning

garment, take the time to consider whether the clothes are still appropriate, and you think they are still stylish.

Sometimes you will have clothes that are just mistakes. Maybe you spent a lot of money on them (or not enough), maybe they were gifts from special people or remind you of special times. Sometimes you just don't wear them but aren't sure why. But to be blunt, if you aren't going to wear them, they are a waste of your closet space. If you already know that you won't wear it just put it in one of your disposal boxes. Or if the clothes are *very* special, make arrangements for proper long term preservation and conservation. As you do this, try to identify what is "wrong" with them and note it in your book. Understanding what you don't like will help you to make better purchasing decisions in the future.

If it doesn't fit get rid of it. If it's too big you don't want it there giving you permission to size up. If it's too small, and you know in your heart of hearts you really aren't going to slim down, donate it. (And if you do slim down, you can celebrate with new clothing!) If you love it, but think it would benefit from lengthening or shortening, changing buttons or trim then put it in the tailoring box, make a note in your book and set a date to get it done by.

Your skin and/or hair colour may have changed, or you may have undertaken a colour consultation so take the time to assess whether the colour of clothing still suits you and you still like it. If you can't see that it works in the mirror, try the magazine spread technique I mentioned in Step Three (Establish Your Style). If it doesn't work, donate it.

If you can, try to identify at least one garment that is the perfect colour - you can wear this when you go shopping as an easy colour comparison test for potential purchases.

As you allocate each item to its new home, check the pockets. At worse, you might find old tissues, but at best there might be money or jewellery you had forgotten about.

4. Clean Your Storage Spaces

Re-imagine your closet as a high-end boutique - make the place you store your clothes a clean, pleasant and relaxing place to be in. Sweep the floors and dust the shelves.

Think about whether you would like to redecorate your boutique by repainting or applying wallpaper. If you feel you need better lighting but don't want to pay for additional electrical installation, consider installing a battery-powered light.

Ask yourself if the storage is adequate; would you prefer to dispose of more clothes or add more storage? You could add double hanging rails so that you can see your tops positioned above your bottoms. Add pretty racks, boxes and baskets for storage. If you don't already have one, get a full-length mirror so that you can review your outfit before you leave the house.

Buy sets of good quality, solid and supportive (yet attractive) hangers. Make sure that any clips are padded so they don't damage your clothing. Line your shelves and drawers to protect your clothes from splinters.

Maybe include something to deter insects and subtly perfume the space like a Victorian style clove studded orange, cedar blocks, lavender sachets or Savon de Marseille. If you have a large closet you may need several.

5. Refill Your Storage Spaces

Still thinking high-end boutique; neat, clean, easy to navigate.

Put only the clothes that you will wear this season back in the closet. Hang them neatly, facing in the same direction with good air circulation. I prefer one garment per hanger, but if you

Signature Wardrobe Planning

always and only wear this with that, then put them on the one hanger if you prefer that. Fold your clothes and gently put them away.

Depending on what's appropriate for you, you can group your clothes in a variety of ways:

- by colour in order of item, e.g. dresses, pants, skirts, jackets.
- by lifestyle categories, e.g. work, evening, weekend.
- as outfits.

Whichever way you choose, I recommend making sure that the clothes you wear the most often are front and centre of your closet for easy access.

Consider allocating particular items their own drawers (e.g. pyjamas, house t-shirts), and using drawer dividers to keep your small items like socks and underwear organised.

Hang pants from the waist to avoid creased and sagging knees. Support delicate clothing by sewing long loops of tape in the waist to slip over the hanger's hook. You could store them in cotton or bamboo garment bags for added protection.

Place other items where they can be seen:

- hang belts on racks, or the hanger hook of the outfit it goes with. Do not leave them in the belt loops as their weight may stretch and distort the garment.
- hang scarves from a rail.
- choose attractive hooks, racks and/or boxes for jewellery storage.
- store handbags vertically on shelves (like books).

- put shoes on racks or in boxes, with trees where appropriate.

6. Carefully Store Your Off-Season Clothing

If your clothes are ready to wear out of the box, swapping seasons will be much less stressful than if you have to clean and repair everything as it comes out. Even clothes that are not obviously soiled will retain fragrances and body oils that may stain and attract insects.

So set these clothes aside to clean and repair *before* storing them away. Pad them with tissue paper as you fold them, and pack them away in the order that you are likely to want to pull them out (with a natural insect repellent). Store your boxes in a cool dry place out of direct sunlight. If you're lucky enough to have a spare closet, just hang them in cotton or bamboo garment bags (to exclude dust and insects while allowing the air to freely circulate) and swap closets.

You could use moth balls, but they are little balls of concentrated pesticide that work by releasing toxic vapours, and these vapours also soak into your clothes. They are not only toxic when you breathe in the odour but also leave a toxic residue on your skin and this can have serious health implications for some people, particularly children.

According to the Agency for Toxic Substances and Disease Registry, you can minimise your exposure by airing the clothes out for at least 24 hours, ideally outdoors in full sun on a windy day. After this, you should wash them before wearing them.

That sounds like entirely too much drama to me.

7. Shop Your Closet

One last thing before it's over for six months, and that's to build outfits with what is left. You could do this as part of step three (Try Everything On), but you've had a long and hard day, so you might prefer to do this another time when you feel fresh. When you are ready, you can do this in two different ways.

The first is to get washed, style your hair and put on your usual makeup before trying on your clothes again. Start by putting on your first bottom and hold up your first top against it as you look in the mirror. If you do not like the way they look together, put the top back and pick the next one. If you like the way that looks, put it on and try it with all your jackets, other tops, outerwear, accessories, jewellery, scarves, bags and shoes. Note which combinations work, and which require a little something extra. Start again with the third top, and do it all again with the second bottom. Repeat until you have assessed all your bottoms and all your dresses with every other garment.

Alternatively, if you have identified hues, tints and/or shades that work for you, you can compare each garment with everything else without trying it on. You're looking for a comfortable resonance between the colours; if one appears more vivid than another they are not complementarily toned. Once an item doesn't work with one other item, you can discard it because it isn't the right hue/tint/shade to match you or the rest. It's still a good idea to record the combinations that work, and new items to buy.

The advantage of trying things on is that you can see whether the lines and textures are harmonious and whether you can offset any colour irregularities with other items.

SUMMARY

Conduct six monthly reviews that coincide with swapping out your seasonal wardrobe:

1. Get ready: get everything you need together.

2. Gather ALL your clothes together: notice how looking at them makes you feel.

3. Try everything on: assess each item and discard those that aren't right anymore.

4. Clean your storage spaces: think high-end boutique.

5. Refill your storage space: high-end boutique style.

6. Carefully store your off-season clothing: clean and mend them first.

7. Shop your closet: rediscover old friends and decide what new ones you need.

And update your shopping list.

CHAPTER 14

How to Create a Capsule Wardrobe

Capsule is a popular wardrobe term at the moment, but it can be a very confusing concept because the term is used in three very different ways:

1. A small *set* of themed clothes such as summer holidays, work or eveningwear. This concept has also been described as a "clothing cluster" and a "clothing unit", but for ease of comparison I'm going to call this a cluster.

2. The *basis* of your wardrobe - a small core collection of good quality clothing, supplemented by "extras", that meets your daily needs for four or five years. Variants include the "ten item wardrobe", or if you are hard core the "five item wardrobe". I'm calling this a capsule.

3. Your *complete* wardrobe. This is more of a minimalist approach; each garment is carefully considered according to its appropriateness and stylishness. You only buy it if you

really love it and are prepared to take such good care of it that it will make you happy for a long time. I'm calling this minimalist.

These approaches rely on the same skills and thought processes we discussed in Part Two (Develop Your Wardrobe Plan). Regardless of which approach you choose, you still need to know what clothes are appropriate and stylish for you if you want it to succeed. Ideally you would conduct a wardrobe review (see previous chapter) before you change your approach and build your new wardrobe from there.

While I discuss them separately, given the thought you have already put in, there is no particular reason why you can't combine approaches. For example, if you live somewhere cold develop a capsule wardrobe supplemented by an outerwear cluster. Or an eveningwear cluster if you attend a lot of functions. Or whatever else is a significant need for you.

I think that any of the personality types can use any of these approaches, but I think each will be more drawn to one than the others. For example, the type one probably won't want to use just one approach, but a two might prefer carefully planned clusters. The three might prefer a capsule so they can just get dressed and get going, whereas the four might choose the minimalist approach.

Regardless of that, pick the one that makes sense to you, and give it a go.

The Cluster Method

The cluster method offers you the option of creating a large and varied wardrobe over time, and depending on how you put them together, each cluster offers the start of the next.

In general, each cluster contains five to twelve items in colours that flatter you and can be mixed and matched to create a number of outfits. It is not necessary that each garment matches every other garment, but it should work with at least three others. A mixture of prints and plains in all season fabrics offers the most versatility. You should try to avoid buying standalone and duplicate items, and buy "classic" styles.

Each cluster requires a set of accessories, which according to your needs could include:

- minimum two pairs of shoes - simple tailored and dressy in your clothing colour
- hosiery the same tint as your skirts
- handbag the dominant colour of the cluster
- scarves that complement the cluster, perhaps in your accent colour
- good quality belts 1" - 2" (2 - 4 cm) wide
- simple watch with a plain band
- two pairs of earrings - simple metal and pearl
- two necklaces - simple metal and pearl
- classic chain or bangle bracelet

Your first cluster starts with two main colours that look good together, and an idea of what lines or shapes you want to use. Depending on what's left in your closet, your colours could come from an existing garment or if you are starting afresh, something like a new scarf.

Here's an example of how to put together an eleven piece cluster with a 48 outfit capacity:

- two jackets; dark and either patterned (e.g. herringbone) or a lighter colour

- three bottoms; to match jackets and tops

- four tops; your version of white, light, patterned, and an accent colour

- two sweaters; plain cardigan to match tops and bottoms and a V or jewel neck pullover that can be worn alone or with tops. The pullover should fit under the cardigan and jackets.

Or if you prefer dresses, five (colour blocked, light, small pattern, neutral, pattern or accent) with two jackets and/or cardigans (different colours and styles that match all the dresses) for fifteen outfits.

Once you have completed your first cluster, you can start building a second in a different colour combination. According to the limits of your budget, and need for variety you could create a completely new and separate cluster, build a semi-separate cluster based on one or two items from your first, or expand your existing cluster by incorporating another colour.

The Capsule Method

According to this method, a well-chosen capsule will supply an outfit for every possible occasion. This version includes:

1. plain jacket in a textured fabric - the texture makes it obvious that it is not part of a suit

2. plain skirt in a durable all season fabric in a complementary colour that matches the lines and detailing of the jacket

3. plain pants that can be worn for day and eveningwear that match the jacket

4. minimum two blouses in a size, shape, colour and style that is appropriate for you

Signature Wardrobe Planning

5. simply styled sweater with round neck in the same or complementary hue/tint to the jacket

6. slightly longer than knee length raincoat in a neutral colour. It should protect you from the wind and rain, and be big enough to wear over your jacket, but not so big that you swim in it wearing the dress (see below)

7. if you can afford it, a dark coloured mid-calf coat in a durable and warm fabric.

8. simple dress, appropriate for your lifestyle, that you can dress up or down

9. two pairs of shoes - chunky heel for pants and delicate for dress and skirt

10. minimum three sets of hosiery - sheer black, opaque black and skin tone

11. jewellery - discreet earrings - small pearl studs and small metal hoop or studs

12. scarf to bring colour into your outfit, and protect your jacket from your makeup

13. good quality bag in a size and shape that is appropriate and stylish for you

14. good quality watch in a size and shape that is appropriate and stylish for you

15. good quality gloves in a neutral colour and style; lined if you need extra warmth

16. good underwear that fits snuggly, but not too snuggly

17. minimum two belts, 1" (2 cm) and 2" (4 cm) wide in a classic style to match your shoes or outfit - the buckle should match the jewellery you wear the most often (gold or silver)

Ideally, your eveningwear could be drawn from this capsule (except for very formal occasions). Generally this would be your jacket with the skirt, pants or dress and appropriate and stylish accessories.

If you don't think this prescription works for you, or you are a 20% dresser consider the ten (or five) item wardrobe. This small number tends to freak people out, but think of these core items as being like your family, with other additional pieces (extras) being your friends - if chosen well, your friends will fit in with your family for a long time.

Your ten core items will generally be your middle layers (like dresses, jeans, and tops) supplemented by extras; your under and outer layers and accessories. So your wardrobe will be as big or small as you need. For example, your two dresses, three bottoms and five tops will be supplemented by underwear, coat, cardigan, shoes, accessories, gym clothes and eveningwear according to your needs. Or if you prefer to wash your clothes less frequently you might pick four dresses, six bottoms and ten tops (or two, six and twelve for example).

THE MINIMALIST APPROACH

The minimalist approach, is minimalist in the sense of a small wardrobe, it doesn't *require* the same sort of neutral colour focus that a capsule wardrobe might. Though if you like neutrals, wear them happily.

Have you seen (or do you remember being) a child dancing with impatience, waiting for their favourite outfit to become available for wearing? Or having it scraped off for washing (tantrums notwithstanding) because they didn't want to stop wearing it? The minimalist approach aims to get that feeling of wearing your favourite clothes every day. If you absolutely adore your lime green beaded parakeet top then wear it frequently; to work, to the supermarket, wherever it makes you happy.

Logically, this means you need at least one outfit for each of the activities you identified when you were determining what was appropriate for you. And of course, your style determines how many pieces each of those outfits require. And this determines how many clothes you need.

If you aren't exactly sure how to start, you could begin with something like the Project 333 method developed by Courtney Carver. Choose only 33 items of street wear (including jewellery, shoes and other accessories) for the next three months. The 33 doesn't include your gym clothes, underwear and other house clothes like pyjamas and leisurewear. Like the ten item wardrobe, 33 is a random number that will work for most but not all people. It needs to be tailored to meet your requirements for appropriateness and stylishness.

SUMMARY

A capsule wardrobe is different for everyone. The common approaches are:

- clusters of mix and match clothes
- a capsule of items (family) supplemented by extras (friends)
- minimalist buying and wearing only what you love

Knowing which approach is right for you helps you determine how many clothes you need.

CHAPTER 15

What Good Fit Looks Like

Style is a reflection of who you are, and to an extent that is based on your physical size and shape. When you wear clothes that fit correctly you will feel more comfortable and more confident. And when your clothes fit your body in the right places, you will look good because your clothes are not hinting at figure flaws that aren't there.

Like everything else about you, your shape is not fixed but changes according to your lifestyle and stage of life. That doesn't just relate to your age, but to your menstrual cycle as well. On average, women gain and lose between one and six pounds (450g - 2.7kg), and some as many as ten (4.5kg) over the course of their cycle. (You might want to mention this when you get fitted for a bra - and the best time to get fitted is the week after your period). Not to mention other conditions that may prevent a stable weight and body shape/size.

And just to make things even more difficult, despite what we have come to think of as "standard sizes" they are not standard at all. Each brand has its own version of the size, and very often its own numbering system as well. And just when you get comfortable with that brand, you are squeezed out of its target demographic and can't find anything to fit anymore.

If that is not complicated enough for you, add in "generous", "relaxed", "classic" and "trim" fits. As well as "boyfriend", "skinny" and "super skinny" fits. Throw in some "high", "mid" and "low" rises. Or "loose" and "slouchy". I could go on and on.

While good fit rises from your body shape and Greek Proportions, what you think is a good fit also depends on your fashion personality's toleration for the tightness or looseness of your clothes. For example, personality type one wants clothes that feel light and fresh, the two soft and loose, the three dynamic and sexy, and the four structured and fitted.

But there are some practical requirements for ease of movement that determine what makes a good fit as well. Some fashion seasons are going to be more difficult than others for you to stay true to your ideas of stylishness.

Breasts

Ideally, your breasts will appear to sit equidistant between your waist and shoulders. They have very little in the way of built in support structure and will droop as the decades pass. If you would like to keep them perky as long as possible, you need a bra that offers good support and minimises bounce. A fitting at a lingerie store will help you choose a good supportive bra that does this. They can also help you select bras that minimise or maximise your assets if that's what you want.

Signature Wardrobe Planning

WAISTS

While I disagree with the notion that you need to dress to "balance" your figure, knowing whether you are long or short waisted can help you identify where your lines should be.

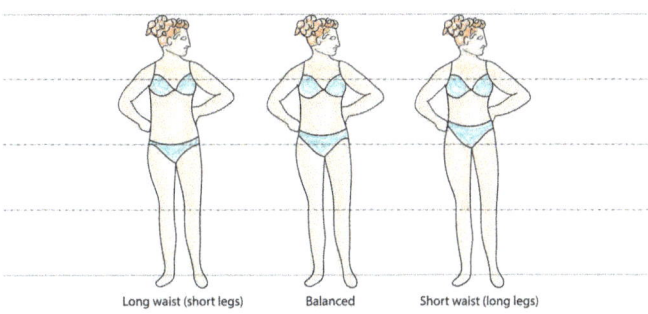

Figure 5: Long, Balanced and Short Waists

Long Waist: if the distance between your shoulders and waist is longer than your waist to the floor (short legs), then your body's proportion is 75% up top and 25% down below. You will probably find that tops and jackets are too short, and tops come untucked. Your pants may be way too long and need tailoring. You might find that the proportional fit "tall" tops and "petite" bottoms work well for you.

Balanced: if the distance between your shoulders and waist is more or less the same as your waist to the floor, your body's proportion is 50% - 50%. You won't have any problems with lengths, but might find it hard to create curves.

Short Waist: if the distance between your shoulders and waist is shorter than waist to floor (long legs), your body's proportion is 25% - 75%. Depending on your personality type, you might find that your ready-to-wear clothes make you feel fat and frumpy because your tops don't lie flat at your waist, your jackets don't sit nicely, your shaped waists hit your hips and your darts are in all the wrong places. You might find the "petite" tops and "tall" bottoms better.

Again, your personality type will influence how you manage your waists. For example:

- type one might be wearing a flirty little dress that should be fitted above the waist and flared out under, and depending on the dress this may or may not bother you.

- type two is probably wearing a loose unstructured dress so this may not concern you at all.

- A young type three might lean in the direction of type one or if older in the direction of type four.

- type four will probably be wearing something fitted and want the waist of your dress to be in the same place as your body's waist.

Alternatively, you could adopt (the proportionally correct) empire or dropped waist as a signature and avoid the waist conundrum altogether.

Hips

The hips anchor skirts and dresses because they are generally shaped and curved according to that measurement. Your hip and the garment hip should sit at the same place; too high and the garment pouches around your waist and/or lower back, too low and it restricts your leg movement and hangs weirdly.

General Fit Issues

It doesn't matter what size you are, you will always look shapelier and better dressed in clothes that have some shape.

Clothes that skim your body do not make you an attention whore, or a tease, they just demonstrate that you care enough about yourself and others to dress well. Embrace your curves!

Conversely, you will always look lumpy and lazy in clothes that are too big or too small. As I mentioned, the number on the label bears no relevance to whether a garment fits or not. It is unlikely that there is even one single ready-to-wear garment out there that is a perfect fit for you - they are manufactured to fit the maximum number of bodies possible. You will only get a perfect fit by having individual items tailored to fit.

When you try clothes on, take three sequential sizes of each garment so that you can gauge the fit, and pick the ones that fit your hips or breasts the best.

The way to do this is to try moving in the way that you would expect to when you wear the garment. For example, if it's a business suit, sit, walk, reach for a file on a shelf, bend to pick something up and so on. Or if it's for a gala event, sit, dance, visit the bathroom, and so on. (It's quite tricky mimicking all that in some small fitting rooms...).

If the garment gives you the freedom of movement you require it's a very good start. And if you can get dressed without someone else's help, then that's even better.

You should have plenty of room for arm and shoulder movement, skirts should not pull up significantly when you sit. The seams at shoulder, neck, underarm and waist should correspond with their body parts.

Clothes that are too tight will restrict your movement, reduce your efficiency and make you feel uncomfortable:

- They should be uniformly snug, including an allowance of looseness to allow for comfort when standing and sitting. They should balance on the body and suggest its contours.

- The main fit problem is shaping flat fabric to rounded surfaces. Garment design lines should be placed on the body contour lines related to the joint articulation to reduce interference, e.g. shoulder seams should sit at the shoulder.

- The fabric's crosswise threads (weft) must be parallel at chest, bust, hip and arm hole while the lengthwise threads (warp) are perpendicular to them and parallel to the centre front.

Almost every single fit flaw can be corrected with a tiny seam lift or drop to gather in or release a little fabric. Even older clothes that are still in good condition can be altered to fit your changing shape. The lesson here is to make your clothes fit your body, not to make your body fit your clothes.

If you can't quite get your head around this concept, put a t-shirt on back to front to give yourself an idea about the difference in the shape of each side of your body and how the shirt has been constructed to fit the shape.

Most of these tweaks are unachievable for someone who doesn't understand dressmaking or tailoring, so while I have mentioned that clothing can be adjusted it's best to start your new relationship with a dressmaker/tailor with some simple adjustments like hems before progressing to more difficult ones. An expensive garment rendered unwearable by poor alterations is a double loss (been there too).

Learn More

You can learn about fit in general by looking at vintage photos, and seeing how the shapes, lines and trims divide the body. Kind of like a geometry problem or colouring book. Clothes from the 1930s to the 1950s were generally very flattering for women's bodies, and vintage images are more likely to accurately represent the shape of the woman wearing them. As you look, also notice how the changes in fashion and manufacture have affected the closeness of fit.

You can get a better idea of what good fit might look like on your body by looking at what similarly sized women are wearing and analysing the fit. You have to do this in real life - Photoshop was invented in 1987, and is so prevalent that it is unlikely that you will see a still or moving image that hasn't been altered in some way - even mine in the back of this book (wish my skin looked that good). Any image can be converted into a digital format for manipulation. There are also old school tricks like pinning excess fabric at the back of a garment to produce a closer fit; you should be suspicious of almost every single modern image you are exposed to.

As you observe live women, bearing in mind the different personality types, ask yourself whether you think her clothes look too tight (does it look like she is about to split her clothing skin)? Or are they too loose (would she benefit from a little more shape in the clothes)? How do you think the shape and fit could be improved?

Once you have developed this knowledge, you will be in a better position to accurately assess your own fit, by feel *and* look. As I mentioned, you need to try the garment on in several sizes, and not fixate on the number - it doesn't mean anything. And you need to look at your whole self, not just the bits you don't like.

JACKETS

Most women will wear a jacket of some description almost all the time; for warmth, to hide "figure flaws", to set boundaries, to increase credibility or for dress codes. They may be the hardest working clothes you have and if they don't fit well they will ruin your carefully constructed outfit.

Buy it to fit either your bust or hips, whichever is largest and have it tailored to fit. If it feels tight when you fold your arms across your chest, and/or the last button doesn't lie flat over your hips it is too small and you need to go up a size and have it taken in at the back. Keep the shoulder pads in proportion to your body not in fashion.

Proportionally speaking (as opposed to fashionably) the most flattering length is to your leg break - the strangely interesting Ancient Greek line. The best fit skims your body but is sufficiently loose to allow a full range of movement.

It should easily button over your breasts without gaping, and collars should lie flat. The shoulder should be 1/4" - 1/2" (0.6 - 1.27 cm) wider than your top, and the sleeves end at your wrist bone allowing the 1/4" - 1/2" (0.6 - 1.27 cm) of blouse to show. The waist should sit at your natural waist.

Skirts

Buy skirts to fit the largest of your waist or hips, and have them tailored to fit. In terms of proportion, around knee length is usually best (strangely interesting again).

A well-constructed skirt will have straight seams that don't permit any sagging around your bottom, and the hemline will be straight and parallel to the floor. While fashion may dictate asymmetric hems, they should still have a geometric consistency to them that is parallel to the floor, for example, an asymmetric hem that sits at a 45° angle to the floor. A good fit will allow you to comfortably get two fingers under the waist, and pinch an extra inch (2.5 cm) at the hip. Vents and pleats should lie flat and not gape.

Pants

Similar to skirts, buy to fit the largest of your waist or hips, and have them tailored to fit. You should be able to comfortably get two fingers under the waist, but pinch an extra 2" - 3" (5 - 7.5 cm) at the hip. The extra fabric allows some give when you sit and goes some way to concealing panty lines. Pleats and pockets should lie flat and not gape, and the crotch should be comfortably loose. The leg crease should fall straight, and the pants should NOT be shaped to fit your bottom. Ideally, the front of the hem would just skim the top of your shoe, though some prefer the back of the hem to fall longer at the heel.

Tops

Tops should be long enough to stay tucked in when you move. Darts should point towards the nipple and stop within 1" (2.5 cm) of it. The neckline should not wrinkle or gape, nor the front of the bust. The sleeve should sit at the shoulder, where the bone pivots when you raise your arm to the side.

Sleeve lengths can be as long or short as you are comfortable with, so long as they allow good freedom of movement and are proportionally correct for you. It's a good idea to try them on with your outfit, particularly the jacket you will be wearing it with to ensure it sits well around the neck.

Sweaters

As they are stretchy, they are often bought too small and therefore too tight. The armhole should not be too tight, and the sleeves should fit over the wrists.

Dresses

Dresses come in a wide variety of styles so it's difficult to lay down guidelines. The easiest way to deal with them is to think of them as a top with a skirt and follow both those guidelines.

Underwear

Correctly fitted underwear smooths out lumps and bumps and supports the body in an upright and dignified stance (they should assist good posture). It should be snug, but not too snug. I recommend a proper bra fitting at a proper corsetiere or lingerie store.

Shoes

Shoes should fit well and comfortably; it is impossible to look or feel beautiful or confident when your feet hurt.

Like clothes, shoes come in brand variants of standard sizes. A well fitted shoe will be at least 1/2" (1.27 cm) longer than your foot when standing, and wide enough that it does not cut off your circulation. The toe box should be wide enough to allow your toes to lie flat, and the inside line of the shoe should be straight, following the line of a normal foot. The widest part of the shoe should fall at the big toe joint, while fitting snuggly at the heel and instep. The shank should be flexible unless extra support is required.

Most manufacturers restrict the number of widths available, so if a shoe is tight across the foot, you may need to go up a size and use an insole to prevent the shoe stretching across the foot and the toe from curling. Those with thin feet will be better to try a specialist shoe store for narrow fittings because shoes that are too wide will continually slip off.

Your feet will change size and/or shape over your lifetime, so *every* time you buy a pair of shoes make time for a fitting.

Generally each manufacturer uses its own version of a three-dimensional foot for a mould (known as a last) and they are usually consistent across all sizes. So when you try on a shoe that just doesn't work for you, it is unlikely that any of that brand's styles will work. However, when you find a shoe that does work, there is an excellent chance that all the brand's other shoes will work for you too.

Summary

When your clothes fit well you look polished. A good fit is indicated by a uniformly unrestrictive level of snugness. You will not get a perfect fit when you buy ready-to-wear clothing, but must buy the best possible fit and have the garment tailored to fit well. Understanding this will save you from fitting room depression, and help you to decide whether to purchase a garment or not.

CHAPTER 16

What Good Quality Looks Like

The very first thing to mention is that price does not necessarily indicate good quality. Sometimes expensive things are poorer quality than inexpensive things. The next thing is that designer or big brand names do not necessarily indicate good quality either, sometimes no names or emerging designers provide better quality.

A good quality garment, let's say a sweater, is one that fulfils the requirements of its form and function - it looks good and keeps you warm. It will almost always fit well, be made from durable materials that are appropriate for the garment's purpose, and sufficiently well made to survive many washes without losing its shape.

Having said that, I have to acknowledge that good quality is not a fixed thing, it changes according to your circumstances. The key measure is the extent that they meet *your* needs and are fit for *your* purposes.

Quality changes according to your budget, which is why you are often advised to buy the best quality you can afford. Perhaps right now you can only afford acrylic sweaters and aspire to wool blend, or maybe you have merino and aspire to a cashmere blend.

It also changes according to what's appropriate for you. If you live in a colder climate, acrylic sweaters are probably not going to work for you so you may have to start with wool. If you are also allergic to wool you will have to work with one of the more recently developed synthetic fleeces.

And it also relates to your style. If you are a personality type three or four, you probably prefer practical and durable clothing and think that a good quality garment should last for several years in which case you might prefer a densely woven single colour wool sweater (that you are prepared to take good care of). If you are type one, you probably prefer constant variety and might think a good quality garment should be exhausted in six months and consequently choose something brightly patterned with a high synthetic content that can be thrown in the washing machine and worn the next day.

I think that a good quality garment has to have an amount of flexibility about it as well. Flexibility in the sense of multipurpose; something you can dress up or down. Something that looks like a whole other thing depending on what else you wear it with, for example, necklace or scarf.

There is a vast difference between a well-made garment and one that is not. Do not buy a garment that is not well made because you will not feel comfortable or well dressed in it. You won't wear it and it will be a waste of your budget. And why would you let someone cheat you like that anyway? YOU deserve well-made clothing, refuse to settle for anything else.

FABRICS

It was once relatively easy to determine whether a fabric was reasonable quality or not by how it felt. Most clothing is now manufactured offshore and shipped back, so they are treated with chemicals to deter pests and maximise the number of clothes per packing unit (this is why you should always wash new clothes before you wear them). These chemicals affect the hand feel so that in some cases clothes feel more luxurious than they are, and in others flaws and unevenness in the weave and construction are concealed.

Most fabrics are either woven or knitted, and the manufacture should be firm and regular with no variations, and a good balance between the threads. Loose weaves and knits are more prone to shrinkage than tight. Irregular yarns (often visible) can lead to breakages and yarn slippage may result in stretching. Modern fabrics are commonly preshrunk before they are made into clothing, but it is always a good idea to follow the care instructions to minimise further shrinkage.

Designs may be part of the weave/knit, either from coloured threads (e.g. checked gingham) or as extra threads woven in to create a pattern (e.g. dotted swiss cotton). Or they can be dyed and/or printed on the completed fabric though in some cases these processes can damage it, and reduce its durability.

If you are familiar with a fabric's characteristics you can get an idea of the amount of treatment that may have taken place and make a decision about whether to purchase the garment. You might find it useful to visit a good vintage clothing store or one that sells bulk fabric to see what they look and feel like (though the fabric bolts will have some treatment as well):

Silk should glisten and hang in soft folds. When you scrunch it the fabric will hardly crease. It feels soft and can be squashed into a small and compact space. Generally rubbing the fabric between your fingers will not affect its finish except in weaves like satin. The fibres are usually long and straight and difficult to pull apart.

Artificial silks (rayon and acetate) will drape like silk but crease a lot when scrunched. They can be manufactured into a number of finishes, so it's not really possible to generalise on the hand feel, the effects of running or breaking.

Wool is dull and heavy, and when scrunched it will bounce back barely creased. It feels warm and springy, especially in a silk blend, but stiffer with cotton. Wool may roughen on rubbing, which may indicate recycled fibres though some blends will not show any effect. The fibres are a little rough and a bit wavy, and can be pulled apart.

Cotton is dull and foldable; when scrunched it will stay creased. It is generally smooth, but when rubbed you might find that the fabric appears thinner and there may be some residue on your fingers. The fibres are short, but if spun well, somewhat difficult to break.

Linen has a little shine, and can be folded but scrunch creases will persist. It comes in a variety of weaves and finishes, but generally you can feel some texture, and when new it might feel cold. It is similar to cotton in that the fabric may appear thinner and leave residue on your fingers. Linen is usually made of very long threads that are difficult to break.

If you can, look at some sewing pattern books to see if you can understand how the finished items are constructed from the illustrations, and maybe why they recommend the fabrics that they do:

- **Appearance:** not just the pattern and colour, but also the texture. A very smooth texture suggests careful handling is needed and may be most suitable for eveningwear, rougher and sturdier suggests suitability for more physical activities.

- **Durability:** can withstand wear and tear, and cleaning without losing shape or colour

- **Comfort:** smooth and soft, or light and cool, or even warm and snuggly.

These things are all characteristics of quality, but they are not all equally important; most people will think comfort is the most important characteristic of quality in their underwear. Overall, the construction worker may favour durability whereas the lawyer might prefer appearance. Comfort may be the most important consideration for your winter clothes, but the comfort you value in your sweaters is not the same kind of comfort you value in your overcoat.

Ready-to-Wear Clothing

When reviewing the quality of ready-to-wear clothes, you should firstly consider the information already covered on fabric quality. Do not be afraid to touch the clothes, to assess the feel by gently rubbing, scrunching and pulling the fabric.

In general, the design of the fabric will be suitable for the garment, that is, the pattern does not conceal the lines of the garment or vice versa. For example, a tartan (plaid) looks best in an unbroken expanse, a detailed garment line made of godets and yokes is best made from a plain fabric that suits tailoring. Pants should be made from a firm fabric that suits a tailored appearance. Tops should be in keeping with the outfits they go with - dressy with dressy, tailored with tailored, and so on.

Higher quality garments are generally well constructed. Inspect the garment to ensure these indicators of skilled manufacture are present.

- The seam allowances are a minimum 5/8" (1.6 cm) to permit alterations if necessary.

- If the garment is shorter than you like, that the hem allowance is large enough for you to lower it.

- The seams are straight and do not drift diagonally off course.

- The pieces are all assembled with the grain in the same up/down direction (when you look across the fabric there are no inconsistencies in the sheen or texture).

- Areas of wear such as the neck and sleeve edges are reinforced.

- Collar edges and corners are slim and flat.

- Zippers are sewn in with matching thread, the stitching is straight and not puckered, and that the zip opens and closes smoothly.

- The stripes and tartans match at major seams.

- The top stitching matches or contrasts with the garment and is even and not puckered.

- You can't see the hem stitching from the right side.

- The button holes are smooth, evenly stitched with no loose threads, and the buttons are securely attached (on a shank if the fabric is thick).

- The pleats, vents and pockets are stitched closed to prevent damage in store (you should remove these when you are ready to wear the garment as they permit ease of movement).

Signature Wardrobe Planning

- That the left and right sides of tops and jackets are the same length.

- The lining fabric complements the garment and is not visible from the right side.

- The darts are stitched well and don't pucker.

- The seams and button holes of thin sweaters are reinforced with tape to prevent stretching.

Conversely, poor quality garments are generally not well constructed.

- seams have small or no allowances
- seams are puckered
- collars are puckered and/or do not lie flat
- the teeth of hidden zippers are visible and/or the stitching is puckered
- stripes and plaids aren't matched
- crooked stitching
- the hem is visible and/or puckered on the right side of the garment
- button holes are not closely and evenly stitched, and/or buttons have loose threads
- left and right sides of tops and jackets are not the same length

SHOES

A good quality shoe will comfortably balance and support your weight on a well-placed heel. It should be well made, and if cared for, last for several seasons. A poor quality shoe is uncomfortable and can cause foot deformities including corns, hammer toes and bunions.

Summary

Quality is a personal thing that varies according to your budget, what is appropriate for you, and what your style is. A good quality garment fulfils its form and function and is well made from flawless fabric that is suitable for its purpose.

CHAPTER 17

Decoding Dress Codes

Dress codes rise from an assortment of sumptuary laws that governed what sorts of clothes could be worn by what sort of people. This included things like the Ancient Roman restrictions on who could wear togas and the width and colours of their stripes, or the styles of vestments worn by different ranks of medieval priests, and the restriction of purple and ermine for royalty.

These laws relaxed and lapsed over time, leaving vestiges like the White Tie code which is still strictly regulated today. Other codes developed as ways of differentiating groups of people, for example the courtroom dress differences between barristers and the judicial hierarchy in some countries.

For most people, the main time they will be confronted by a dress code will be for an event, when getting dressed up will be the most exciting and confusing of things. The most formal is the white tie (which most of us will never be invited to) with relaxing expectations and greater freedom of expression as you work your way down to casual. Regardless of the situation, remember to dress your version of stylish.

The following list includes not just commonly requested codes like black tie, but the strange and unexpected codes that sometimes come up, and common situations where you might find yourself at a loss for what to wear. It is in alphabetical order just to make it easier to navigate.

Aeroplane Travel

This is a tricky one, particularly on a long-haul flight because you need to be comfortable. Your clothes should be made from natural fibres so your body can breathe, and not restrict your circulation (you don't want deep vein thrombosis).

You should wear comfortable shoes, and bearing in mind that some airport security checks may require you to remove them, something like ballet flats or loafers would be best. If you have any kind of fluid retention issues consider compression tights or leggings rather than just socks.

If you'd like to be upgraded you need to look the part. Wear dressy/smart casual; at the very least nice, neat and clean clothes that do not include slogans or pictures that some might think are offensive.

Afternoon Dress

During the late eighteenth and early nineteenth century, you dressed for the time of the day not the event; informal in the morning, more formal as the day passed. Afternoon dress was semi-formal for making and receiving callers at home (as opposed to meeting in public at an event). It occasionally comes up as a suggested code at events like Royal garden parties, and appropriate attire is still in the semi-formal range.

See also Morning, Semi-Formal and Tea Dress.

Black Tie

Also known as morning dress, a slightly less formal dress than the white tie, worn after 6 pm.

- **Men:** a dinner suit (tuxedo), white shirt and black bow tie.
- **Women:** full-length ball gowns in bold colours, best jewellery and heels.

See also Morning Dress.

Black Tie (Creative)

- **Men:** standard tuxedo style, or a fresh interpretation such as a black shirt or red tie.
- **Women:** as for black tie

Black Tie (Encouraged or Optional)

They don't expect you to buy or hire it to wear it to their function, but they would *really* love it if you did. If you don't wear black tie, wear cocktail dress instead.

Business (Casual: Classic)

This relates to what you wear in a more conservative office workplace. It is less formal than the traditional business suit but more formal than casual - you might think of it as a bottom and jacket that don't necessarily have to match. If in doubt, ask to see the dress code.

- **Men:** khaki pants, dark blazer, collared shirt but no tie.
- **Women:** pants or knee length skirt, jacket and high cut collared blouse.

Business (Casual: Relaxed)

This relates to a less conservative office workplace. It is less formal than classic business casual and in some workplaces may include jeans.

- **Men:** khaki pants, polo shirt.
- **Women:** pants or knee length skirt, shell set (twin set).

Business (Formal)

This relates to daytime events like conferences, lunches and so on. It's a dressier version of traditional business dress.

Business (Office Parties)

If it's straight from work in the boardroom, then your usual business attire is acceptable. If it's in a ballroom at a nice hotel then something closer to the cocktail. Just remember it's still work even if it's a party, and you will be seeing these people again at 8 am the next day so dress (and drink) more conservatively than you would at an event with friends and family.

Business (Traditional)

- **Men:** a suit, button down shirt and a tie that matches the shirt.
- **Women:** pant or skirt suit, or professional dress with jacket.

Casual

For most people, merely neat and clean, jeans and sneakers. Whatever! I hope that you will aim higher.

Casual (California, Florida, wherever)

Sort of casual cocktail style - a sort of relaxed elegance but in a cotton dress instead of silk.

Casual (Dressy/Smart)

More relaxed than lounge, but more formal than casual.

- **Men:** pants and blazer, collared shirt, but not necessarily a tie.
- **Women:** separates are acceptable.

NO JEANS ALLOWED!!! Though, just to be confusing, some events interpret dark wash jeans as acceptable (as long as they are not distressed). This code is more of a relaxed formal thing than a formal casual thing.

Cocktail

A semi-formal sort of transition from day to night attire. It arises from the inter-war period when it became common to meet for pre-dinner drinks. It's less regulated than "tie" codes.

- **Men:** dark dress suit (not tuxedo), white shirt and tie.
- **Women:** black, white or jewel-toned knee length dress in a luxurious fabric (with or without beading or metallic effects) bold jewellery and heels. More recently some women prefer to wear a tuxedo.

Dinner Party

Despite being held in someone's home, dinner parties are formal or semi-formal events for adults with invitations and dress codes. Your host will make an extra special effort with the food, so you must make an extra effort with your clothing. A good host will give you an indication of what they expect, like black tie for a "Titanic" event or semi-formal for a coming of age.

Festive (usually related to Christmas)

The code with a festive twist. For example, cocktail could be red and green sequins or casual might be plaid shirts. It doesn't mean festive sweater.

Formal

See Black Tie

Funerals

You probably won't receive dress code instructions, so you may need to do some research to find out what is appropriate for the culture of the funeral you are attending. For example:

- dark conservative clothing is generally expected at Western Christian funerals
- white casual clothing for Hindu
- Japanese have a code called "Hakama" which roughly corresponds to a formal black tie
- you are required to wear a head covering at a Jewish funeral
- you will be required to remove your shoes for a Muslim funeral inside a mosque

You might be asked to wear the deceased's favourite colour, or the colours of their favourite sports team and so on. You might not think this is appropriate and prefer to wear your traditional clothes, but do consider it for the family's sake.

Job Interviews

A lot of this depends on the business you are interviewing with, for example, a law firm will expect a suit, a retail business might expect high fashion and marketing something creative.

However, different jobs have different clothing requirements. If you are interviewing at a law firm for a position in the staff cafeteria, you won't need to dress in a suit like a lawyer, but you will need to be neat and clean. I recommend erring on the side of caution and wearing something like dress pants or khakis and an ironed woven shirt.

You can get ideas by observing the people who work there, and wear something a shade more conservative. Perhaps with a distinctive piece of jewellery to stand out.

It is unlikely that your sweatpants or sheepskin slippers will ever be appropriate interview attire.

Lounge Suit

A little more relaxed than cocktail dress.

- **Men:** neutral suit (e.g. grey or navy) with a tie.
- **Women:** knee length dresses, simple jewellery and heels.

Meeting Potential In-laws

Something a little conservative; highish neckline, longish hem, but still your colours and style. Show them who you are, not what your bits are.

Morning Dress

During the late eighteenth and early nineteenth century, you dressed for the time of the day rather than the event, generally informal in the morning, becoming more formal as the day progressed. Morning dress was plain and informal with high necklines and long sleeves.

More recently the term is used to describe men's Black Tie standards, principally because the informal clothes men wore during eighteenth and nineteenth century mornings are now considered more formal that at that time.

See also Afternoon and Tea Dress.

Mourning Dress

In the West, during the Victorian era there were highly structured and codified expectations about what people who were mourning the death of a close relative should wear. This was partly to protect them from trivialities, and partly to warn others to show some consideration. These expectations have largely lapsed though they persist in some cultures.

If you are in mourning and wish to be left to your own devices, you could try dressing more formally than usual in more structured clothes and darker colours.

Professional

See business

Race Meetings

Horse racing is known as the "Sport of Kings", because it is expensive to raise and train horses. As such, race meetings required very formal clothing (also expensive).

For this reason, older more traditional racing venues require dress closer to the formal end of the spectrum. Many will refuse entry to people dressed casually (jeans, collarless shirts, untailored jackets, sneakers, or flip flops as well as women displaying "excessive" midriff, i.e. belly button).

Hats, by their fleetingly fashionable nature, were once an important indicator of wealth and status, and traditional tracks are likely in insist on a hat or fascinator.

At the absolute minimum, dressy/smart casual will gain entry to an informal track, but lounge will guarantee entry.

Religious Services (e.g. baptism, confirmation, bar/bat mitzvahs, and the like.)

These are generally solemn occasions and require a level of formality in dress for example, high necklines, sleeves, lower hems. However, unlike funerals, they are also celebrations so colours and patterns can be worn.

Like weddings and funerals, the service is often followed by a catered function and these can be a guide to the level of dress required. If you are unfamiliar with the religion, check the expectations about head coverings and shoes are.

School

Naturally something in proportion, harmonious, balanced and in the right colours. In 1949 anyway. Something of simple design, in cotton for summer and wool for winter, perhaps a plain tailored suit with a durable coat, soft hat, lapel pin or wooden bead necklace.

Semi-Formal

- **Men:** dark suit with dress shirt and tie.
- **Women:** somewhere between simple knee length dress, jewellery and low heels and luxurious knee length dress with bold jewellery and high heels.

See also Afternoon Dress

Show (Ballet, Concert, Theatre, Opera)

At one time, the dress code for these events was Black Tie, but it's not unusual to see people dressed very casually (or even in house clothes) at them now. But, as your tickets were probably expensive, and you may not have as many opportunities to dress up as much as you would like, why not dress up a lot. Make an evening of it, and go for drinks or dinner - wear the best outfit that is appropriate for the town that you live in. Lounge suit and up.

Tea Dress

During the late eighteenth and early nineteenth century, you dressed for the time of the day rather than the event, generally informal in the morning, becoming more formal as the day progressed. Tea dress filled the space between morning and afternoon dress; it was also a sort of leisurewear equivalent that you changed into between events to rest and relax in. It was only worn in the company of your most intimate associates and NEVER in public.

See also Morning and Afternoon Dress

Trousseau

This is both a wardrobe of clothes fit for the life of a wife, and the linens (sheets, towels, and so on) she brings to the marriage. Like mourning clothes, it once represented a significant life change, one where unmarried women dressed and behaved differently to wives. Not such a big thing today, though many girls still collect things for their marriages and the bulk are supplied by gifts at showers, engagements and weddings.

WEDDINGS

A dress code will usually be stipulated, and this is generally a more formal level of dress. However, a ceremony in a large public garden followed by a picnic meal will be different to beach ceremony and clam bake, which is again different to a resort hotel or banqueting centre. If in doubt contact your host in the hope that they can be more explicit.

WHITE TIE

The most formal kind of Western dress and nowadays generally only worn after 6 pm at very formal events like State Dinners. It comes with strict requirements about what *must* be worn. As a cheat, think Fred Astaire and Ginger Rogers, but should you ever be invited to a white tie event, make sure you do your homework.

CHAPTER 18

Let's Go Shopping!

Before you go shopping, you need to decide some things. Having developed your basic wardrobe plan as you worked through Part Two (Develop Your Wardrobe Plan), you already know:

1. how much you can spend,
2. what's appropriate for you,
3. what your style is, and
4. what your specific shopping list is.

If you have been working your way through Part Three (Build and Maintain Your Wardrobe), you also have an idea of which characteristics of fit and quality are important to you. Now you just have to decide what your primary shopping goals are. For example, do you want to:

- be the first to wear it, or
- get the best bargain, or

- get it before they run out of your size?

GET READY...

Why You Need to Stick to Your Wardrobe Plan

Writing a detailed shopping list that includes your need, style and budget (pastel pink chiffon ruched sleeveless dress $210), and then sticking to it is the most important part of building your signature look. These details allow you to head directly to the right colour and price point skipping past the temptations of all the others.

You might find it helpful to structure your list as outfits, so that if you can't get one piece you can easily abandon the rest or make an informed choice about whether you can accept any differences and what they are.

Perhaps you will find it easier to think of it as if you were shopping for ingredients for a special meal you hope to cook for someone you care deeply about. If you can't find one of the ingredients that you need, you just can't make that meal. You might be able to substitute some other ingredient, but it won't be quite the same.

Here's an edited example of what can go wrong from spring 1937. The shopping list:

1. warm plain brown wool coat
2. black silk crepe dress and brown suede belt (to wear with coat)
3. black sheer wool dress with wood buttons (to wear with coat)
4. lightweight brown wool jacket (to wear with dresses and skirt)
5. brown/black/white check wool skirt

Signature Wardrobe Planning

6. brown/white patterned silk dress (to wear with or without the coat)

7. brown bag and shoes

8. warm weather essentials - white bag *or* hat plus jacket (to wear with skirt or print dress)

If you didn't stick with the list and instead bought:

1. brown coat with "fur" collar

2. black crepe dress with white trim

3. black wool dress with silver buttons

4. red jacket

5. blue skirt suit

6. black floral dress

you would find yourself with some wardrobe matching, and corresponding cost, quality and wear issues.

- The fur trim makes the coat look too hot for warmer days, and won't be consistent with the floral dress. It will probably look tatty quickly.

- The white trimmed dress will not be consistent with the coat, and the trim will probably discolour unless very carefully washed.

- Silver buttons are very memorable and may reduce the black dress' overall usefulness.

- The red jacket may work with the black dresses but won't match this year's brown shoes.

- The blue suit replaces the check skirt but requires a white bag *and* hat (and savings must be made somewhere else to permit this).

- The black floral dress doesn't match anything else.

- If you go ahead and buy the brown bag and shoes, they won't match your black dresses unless the trims are changed. Nor will they match the floral dress or the blue suit.

- You can't replace the brown bag and shoes with black because they won't match the coat. Nor can you replace with blue as that won't match anything except the blue suit.

- If you buy a cheaper bag and shoe set in both black and blue, they will almost certainly be of poor quality and won't look nice for long.

Many modern designers offer seasonal cluster collections, so if your budget stretches to this, and the clothing meets your needs you may be able to buy your shopping list in one trip.

Otherwise, you need to build on what is already in your wardrobe. This is much easier if you have conducted your wardrobe review (see chapter 13) and know what clothes you have as well as what you want.

Shopping Principles (or Responsibilities)

In addition to the general purchasing principles you created in Part Two (Develop Your Wardrobe Plan), it's worth adding some specifics for your shopping trips. These will help you to make good decisions and reduce stress as you build your signature look and pull your wardrobe together.

1. Follow your wardrobe plan and stick to your budget; no one else cares about them, and paying more for something does require sacrificing something else.

Signature Wardrobe Planning

2. Only buy breathtakingly amazing clothes and comfortable shoes that you want to wear all the time.

3. Don't buy clothes that don't fit, are too conservative or too on trend because you'll never wear them.

4. Wait patiently, and treat sales staff nicely. If you are a pleasure to deal with, it is more likely that they will genuinely help you, offer to order the sizes or colours you want and lay things aside while you think about them.

5. When you get tired and cranky, give up and go home. Start again another day when you are fresh and capable of better decisions.

6. Understand that you have an indirect responsibility for the conditions under which your clothes are produced. Be willing to pay a fair price and require assurances that your clothes have been made in healthy and safe working conditions.

And if you want a gold star, know what your strangely interesting Ancient Greek proportions are, and take a tape measure with you when you shop so that you can measure items out and decide whether you like them enough to try them on (knowing that you will need to alter them to fit properly).

GET SET...

When to Shop

Stores generally have the widest selection of clothing at the turn of the seasons in February/March and September/October. From an efficiency point of view, it may be best to shop twice a year at these times, especially if you need to visit a larger town for your shopping.

I recommend a mad sales dash to pick up your staple socks, underwear and t-shirts followed by a more thorough shop for the rest. I don't recommend buying all of your clothes on sale because you deny yourself the joy of wearing something current while it is still current and you will wear it the most often.

You will make your best clothes shopping decisions when you feel calm and confident. Shopping in the morning when stores are quiet also means that the staff are fresh and may be more helpful, so try to avoid lunchtimes and Saturdays. You could also consider making an appointment to see a personal shopper who can collect together some appropriately stylish clothes for you to try on.

I've already mentioned that standard sizing isn't standard, so give yourself adequate time to try on a garment in a range of sizes, look at them from several angles, and move around in them before making your purchase decision.

Where to Shop

Clothing stores have their own identity, and the window displays are a good indicator of the sort of customer they serve. Each store (regardless of kind) has a target market, so don't be surprised if the sales assistants judge you. While looking neat and tidy in upmarket stores helps a great deal, asking for advice helps a lot more. If the assistant has a good eye and knows their stock well, they will be able to identify clothes that suit you, offer alteration suggestions and maybe recommend a good tailor/dressmaker to undertake them.

However, they may be just as happy to offload the clothes they can't sell to anyone else so listen to your gut, hold hard to your shopping list, and if it doesn't feel right walk away. If the assistant is happy to let you go, it's a reasonable indicator that their opinion can be trusted.

Signature Wardrobe Planning

You can buy clothes that are new and used according to your budget and style.

NEW:

- **Designer Boutiques** stock only the clothes designed under the designer's guidance. They generally design for particular lifestyles so you should start by looking in magazines and advertising to find the ones that design for yours. The clothes will not be cheap, but the stores are worth visiting just to understand the cloth, colour and cut so that you can compare when you get to the department and chain stores.

- **Department Stores** are useful from the point of view that you could probably get everything on your list in one trip, depending on how particular you are. This is quite useful for shopping by outfit.

- **Large Chain Stores** can also fulfil this function, within a smaller range.

- **Discounting/Low-End Department Stores** can be useful for underwear staples and some inexpensive seasonal items.

- **Outlet Stores** once sold end of season clothing at significant discounts, but many stores/designers now design lines specifically for the outlets, providing a cheaper lower quality version of store items.

- **On-line Shopping** is very convenient, but you can't see the garment's true colours, feel their texture or try them on. If it is a brand/designer you know well this can be a relatively stress-free way of shopping, but return postage can become quite expensive and eat up your clothing budget.

- **Catalogue Shopping** is similar to online, but you order from a booklet that comes in the mail. Many stores offer mall, mail and on-line shopping.

- **Trunk Shows** are like Tupperware for clothes and/or shoes. You try on samples, make your order and a few weeks later your clothes are ready for collection. They can be convenient for buying clothing clusters, but may be expensive.

- **TV Shopping Networks** offer fairly effortless shopping in a marginally addictive environment with skilled sales people who make it really easy to overspend if you aren't disciplined.

- **Made-to-measure** by a tailor or dressmaker. You will usually get excellent results, but you will also usually pay significantly for them. The result depends to a large extent on the level of rapport you have with the craftsperson and the quality of the materials they use. You will need to do some research; ask to see samples and reviews.

USED:

- **Consignment Stores** sell lightly worn designer clothes that other people don't want anymore and are hoping to recoup some of the purchase price. They can be a great deal cheaper, but you should check the current retail prices to determine whether you think they are priced sufficiently well. The clothes will be available in limited sizes and may be several seasons old, so if you can't identify what dates them you might be best to skip them. You need to inspect them very carefully to ensure that you are satisfied with the level of wear.

- **Second Hand, Thrift and Charity Stores** offer used clothing (like consignment stores) but more usually everyday clothes in a variety of conditions. They are sold in limited sizes on an as is basis (no exchange) and need to be inspected carefully before purchase.

NEW AND USED:

- **On-line Auctions** offer a great opportunity for fabulous purchases as well as a tremendous disappointment when goods turn out to be unsatisfactory. Only buy through sites that offer fraud and buyer protections, and check the seller reviews. Use payment methods that also offer buyer protections such as PayPal or your credit card.

- **Markets** are a great opportunity to buy new and used one of a kind items. You can buy directly from the maker, who often take commissions and sometimes offer choice from a range of fabrics as well.

- **On-line Marketplaces** like Etsy offer vintage clothing and jewellery. Some sellers won't accept returns so check the store policies carefully. Some sellers meticulously document the item condition others not so much, so don't pay more than you are prepared to loose. Etsy also offers handmade clothes direct from the maker, and many will accept commissions as well.

Research Your Shop

Start with reconnaissance. Look in store windows to see what the key looks are: what kind of clothes are matched with which accessories, what colours, what lengths, and what it is that makes them look more current than last year. Then try some clothes on to see whether the colours and styles work for you (take photos if you can't yet see the whole you in the mirror). Take note of things that look better (or worse) than you thought (and why), their full price cost, what you might wear them with and whether you think it might deserve a place in your closet.

Where high-end stores offer an alteration service, it will probably be worth using as they should be familiar with how the clothes are constructed and be able to quickly and easily make the changes. However, for low-end stores this will probably not be the case so you should rely on your preferred tailor/dressmaker instead.

While you are looking around, check for services such as lockers and coat checks where you may be able to store your purchases once you start buying. Also places to sit down and rest for a moment, and wifi hotspots to check your email. You might also want to make a note of your credit card numbers and provider telephone numbers in case your wallet is lost or stolen.

Once you have a good idea of what and where you will be buying, you could prepare a schedule to help you travel the most efficient route to collect it all on the day.

Some people like to work from the cheapest stores up to the most expensive so they can get the best deal, others visit their favourite brands first. Wherever you go, I recommend starting with your most expensive items and working down to the cheaper ones so that you are making your best decisions about your most significant purchases when you are fresh.

Go!

The Day(s) of the Shop

Wear comfortable clothes and shoes that you can easily take off and put on. If you have something in a colour you love and know looks good on you wear it so that you can test potential purchases against it - if the colour of the new garment sits nicely with it, it's going to be fine but if one seems more vivid than the other they are different shades/hues/tints and won't harmonise so you can put it back without trying it on.

Make sure your underwear is appropriate (everyday if shopping for everyday clothes, fancy for good) so that you can check bra and panty line coverage. Do not wear sports bras unless you are shopping for active wear because they are generally enormous and you won't get an accurate idea of coverage.

It can also be useful to wear the appropriate makeup to see how the outfit colours and patterns balance your face. Does your everyday red lipstick overwhelm the garment or do you need stronger colours on your face because the garment washes you out?

The clothes that you are looking for are potential additions to your existing collection, so bring (or wear) the shoes and accessories you are trying to match with you. But not so much that it's going to kill you carrying them around (hopefully your reconnaissance identified lockers).

Consider bringing water and small snacks as well - it's going to be a big day. Or not - I prefer to sit and take a breather now and then, and if there is wifi, coffee and cake that's all good.

Do your shoe shopping at the end of the day when your feet have swollen, and try them on with appropriate socks or hosiery (e.g. hiking socks for hiking boots and stockings for pumps). Fit to your biggest foot, which is usually opposite to your writing hand. Wriggle your toes and walk about. It *is* possible to buy a pair of shoes that are comfortable and do not need to be stretched or worn in, so if you go up a size and they are still excessively uncomfortable, don't buy them.

As the day progresses, it will become more and more tempting to just buy any old thing. If you start feeling that way, give yourself permission to stop shopping and go home without buying another thing. If you buy things that you think will probably do, you will either never return them or will waste your precious time and effort returning them. Or even worse, force yourself to wear them and feel uncomfortable knowing all along that they are just not right.

What to Look for When you Try Clothes On

As well as considering the information provided in chapter 15 (What Good Fit Looks Like), you need to consider how the garment has been put together.

Before you try anything on, examine the fabric and construction as described in chapter 16 (What Good Quality Looks Like). If the garment meets those requirements, take your three sizes and try them on, hopefully in a good sized fitting room with "daylight" lighting and a triple mirror. Look at garment from all sides.

Cloth:

- Are there any flaws?
- Are the weight, softness, stiffness, and care requirements appropriate?
- Will the texture work with current clothes as well as the purchases you are planning?

Colour:

- Does it suit you?
- Does it make you feel good?
- Will you get tired of it too quickly?
- Will it work with your other clothes?

- Are the trim colours compatible? Will they require special care to maintain?

- Is it too fashionable (or conservative) for the lifespan you expect it to have?

Cut:

- Is it a good fit; are the height and width around the upper arm, the length of the sleeve, the size of the shoulders, chest and hips adequate?

- When you move, do the pleats lie flat? Does the neck or armhole pucker or pull?

- Do the gathers hold sufficient fabric to hang softly? Is the movement appropriate?

- Does it have a flattering shape that is stylistically soft or sharp as you prefer?

- Is it too fashionable (or conservative) for the lifespan you expect it to have?

- Can it be adequately altered?

- Is it comfortable?

Fitting rooms are often small, so don't be afraid to come out for a better look in the big mirror that most stores have in this area - you will get a much better idea of what you look like (rather than the flabby belly and chunky calves).

And there's always the chance a stranger will tell you that you look gorgeous.

SUMMARY

Keep your wardrobe plan to hand and set a shopping goal before you start. Then:

- **Get Ready:** prepare your shopping list and strengthen your resolve to stick to it.

- **Get Set:** research what's in store for the new season; try on clothes in the shapes and colours that are appropriate and stylish for you

- **Go:** Wear comfortable clothes and shop early in the day while everyone is fresh. If you don't love it, put it down and walk away.

CHAPTER 19

How to Choose a Hat

It doesn't matter whether you wear it for warmth, or an occasion, if you're wearing a hat, you'll stand out because they're not common anymore. So, if you're going to wear one, you might as well make it worthwhile.

In some ways, your hat will be a work of art, like a sculpture, with mass, form and line. The line gives it style, and because it's part of an outfit, the line of the hat must be in harmony with the line of the outfit.

The line also speaks about your personality; dramatic, sporty, romantic and so on.

The hat is also part of your head, so it must be in harmony with the lines formed by your face and hairstyle. And in proportion to the size and shape of your head.

You shouldn't look worse in a hat than you do without one. If you do, it's just that you've chosen a hat that doesn't work for you, whether that's the style, or scale, or colour, or texture.

Hat Anatomy

Before we get started, let's take a quick look at what a hat is.

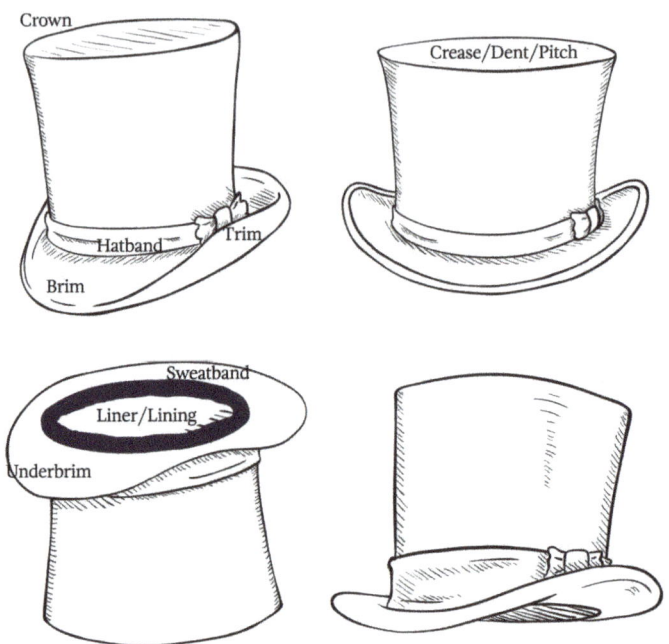

The most common words you're about to read are:
- **Crown:** the top of the hat. The crown may be shaped with a crease on the insde, and dents on the outside. (You'll often see people handling the hat with these in old movies.)
- **Brim:** the bottom part of the hat that protrudes from the crown and shades the face.
- **Trim:** the hat's decoration, commonly a hatband made of ribbon. Sometimes tied in a bow, sometimes beads, buttons, feathers and flowers attached to the band. In some hats the brim may be bound as well

High quality hats usually come with lining and sweatbands to keep the inside clean, and to an extent, stop sweat staining the exterior. If you're planning to wear the hat a lot, it's worth paying extra to get them.

So here's how to choose a hat that works for you.

1. Purpose

Decide what the hat's for.

In the early twentieth century, a woman would generally have a small hat wardrobe. At the very least, it would include an everyday hat for Summer sun protection, another for Winter warmth, and at least one for special occasions.

Regardless of the season, you need to know whether you need formal construction for City work (e.g., Fedora), a durable, practical shape to accommodate Country work like horse riding (e.g., Stetson), or something less formal for leisure.

Will you wear it for hours every day, or for a short while at a special occasion? Is it for work or leisure? Will you wear it for long periods or just a few hours here and there?

These questions help to determine the fabrication and durability you require, and these answers guide you on how much you might be prepared to pay.

2. Budget

You need a hat budget for the same reasons you need a clothes budget; it sets boundaries and makes you think about what you want against what you need.

Technically it's part of your overall clothing budget, and like your clothes, allow more for a hat you'll wear a lot, and less for one you might only wear once or twice.

Like clothes, hats range from cheap mass production to more expensive handmade bespoke hats. The advantage of a custom hat is a better fit for your specific head and hairstyle. An experienced milliner will also make it to suit your body and personality.

To keep costs down, you can get one plain hat and decorate according to your mood, and purchase less expensive materials, such as wool felt instead of fur felt. However, it should be sufficient quality to last a reasonable length of time based on the purchase price.

3. The Outfit Line and Proportion

While most women think first about finding a hat to suit their face, it's more important to match it to your outfit, because it is part of your outfit.

So, choose your winter coat and scarf, or event dress to suit your body. Then take them hat shopping to ensure the shape, colour, texture and balance of the hat results in an overall, well-balanced silhouette or shape.

That's the work of art thing I mentioned at the start of the chapter.

If the outfit is on the plain side of the spectrum, choose a plain hat. Or highly decorative with decorative.

Match the lines of the hat to the lines of your face and outfit. For example, if your coat has rounded collars, choose a hat with a rounded outline on the sides.

Or if your dress has a flared skirt, balance it with a small coronet style hat or a large hat with a drooping brim. Coats with large or (faux) fur collars also balance flared skirts, in which case you'd choose a smaller hat. Or a larger hat if the coat doesn't have a collar.

A large hat generally looks better with a longer skirt than a shorter one. A hat made with velvet will look larger than the same hat constructed in tulle.

It can be difficult and confusing, so make time to look at pictures in old magazines or library archive collections to learn how people used to match it all up.

You may find you prefer certain shapes of hat, and it's possible to get the same shape in a variety of proportions to suit most body shapes. You'll also notice small details, such as hats worn with coats are larger than hats worn with suits or dresses.

Don't forget your glasses! They'll change the size and shape of your face, and you need to make sure the hat can comfortably accommodate them.

4. Age and Position

Just as your clothing needs change over time, your hat needs do too.

As we age, our faces crease and sag and our youthful plumpness relocates to less flattering places.

Depending on your work, you might increase or decrease in dignity, and choose more severe lines, or looser, floppier ones to emphasise the change.

Or to avoid angular lines around your face with a tall, close-fitting turban, or embrace a small, soft hat with a brim that rolls. Or you might prefer a broader brim that casts a shadow over your face, concealing your early wrinkles.

5. Colour and Texture

Now you've chosen a hat with lines to complement your outfit. Next choose a colour that enhances your skin, hair, and eyes, as well as contrasts or harmonises with your outfit. And expresses your style.

Bear in mind the colour will seem different in natural and artificial light, as well as daylight and twilight. And in all conditions, you want the hat to accentuate your good looks, not steal the attention away from you,

You might also like to consider some practicality in the colour. For example, light colours to deflect sunlight or a dark hat that hides the dirt.

Its texture will ideally match your skin and outfit - smooth with smooth (e.g., dresses) and rough with rough (e.g., your winter scarf and coat).

6. FACE

The next step is to look for shapes and textures to complement the lines of your face; a hat's contours, brims, crowns and trim can minimise or emphasise your facial features.

For example, your nose. Drooping or flat brims conceal them, whereas upturned and brimless hats emphasise them, as does centre front trimming. A large brim at the front with a small back can minimise nose size but may exaggerate irregular features.

Or your chin. Folds, drapes, curves and low placed trim around the chin draw attention to it. If you're self-conscious, avoid turbans, pillbox and other small hats. A hat that increases the volume of your upper face, like berets pulled out over the face, can balance a protruding chin.

A medium-sized brim that's wider at the sides, or shows the forehead and focuses on the upper face appears to minimise front heaviness and balances receding chins. Double chins can be minimised with a softly drooping brim, a turn up at the back, or trim that gives the effect of height.

If you're concerned about a thin neck, look for a small soft hat, and skip the severe hats with upturned brims at the back.

Consider rear brims, draped irregular brims, low trim, and curved lines.

Remember, glasses change the size, width, and proportions of your face, so wear them when you're trying hats on. If you don't have a glare reduction coating on your glasses, and want to prevent reflections, choose a turned-down brim.

Soften angular features with round brims and soft edges. Or if you have delicate features, try a classic small brimmed style. Irregular brims generally flatter more than straight, and asymmetric trim distracts from irregularities, while balanced trim can seem to widen the face.

Here are some suggestions for different face shapes, but bear in mind, the shape of your head, the size and shape of your shoulders changes the way people see your face. No two women with the same face shape have the same features.

Heart

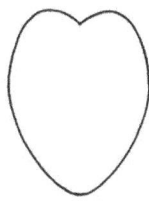

If you have a heart-shaped face and want to balance its perceived roundness, consider avoiding straight brims (e.g., berets and baseball caps, that cut your face in two). Try something asymmetrical with a small brim in a bucket shape, or a smaller brim with off-centre decoration. Avoid wide brims that make your narrow chin look narrower.

Oblong

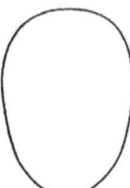

If you're unhappy with the size of your forehead, choose something you can wear forward, or lower to make your face appear shorter. Streamlined shapes with square or round crowns slanted to one side will do well. To balance the width, wear wide crowns, sitting at a slight angle.

Oval

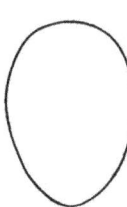

If you'd like to make your face look shorter, try something flared with a wide brim and deep crown like a cloche, pillbox or beanie. Try not to avoid tall hats with a crown narrower than your face.

Pear

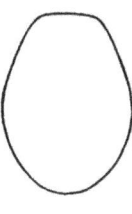

To balance a wide jaw, and draw attention to your eyes, try short, straight or upturned small brimmed styles with high crowns. You could also tuck your hair behind your ears to increase the appearance of width in your upper face. Consider hats with asymmetrical decorative details.

Signature Wardrobe Planning

Round

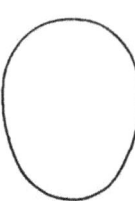

To balance the roundness, avoid straight brims (berets and baseball caps). Choose tidy styles with small brims, worn forward or on a slant to slim the face. Or an upturned brim or high crown gives the illusion of a longer and less round face. Off-centre trim focuses the eye away from the roundness.

Tall, shallow crown will elongate and balance a round the face, as will peaked, slanted, or creased crowns. Brims that are wider than the face make it look narrower by comparison.

Skip the rolled brim.

Square

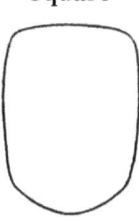

Women with square faces might want to distract from angular features. Large, soft-lined brims, upturned brims, round or curved-edge crowns that soften the face (e.g., cowboy, homburg or cloche) will help.

Hats that sit high on the forehead (e.g., berets or newsboy caps, rounded bowler hats with narrow rolled brims) will lengthen the face. Hats worn on the slant will break up the symmetry.

Beanies might not be the most flattering choice.

Triangle 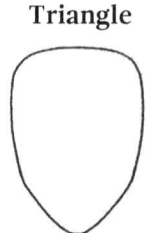 To balance delicate features, wear a smaller brim. Try to avoid a crown narrower than the cheekbones.

Additionally, your hair becomes one with your face, and at the same time, one with your hat.
1. Depending on whether you dress it up or down, or wide at the sides, hair can increase the apparent width and height of your face.
2. It can soften or harden your profile, and exaggerate the size of your features.
3. The size and placement of your hair affects the fit of your hat. Hair that's piled on the top of your head requires a taller crown. A large arrangement at the back of your head requires a deeper fit, and possibly a higher crown as well.

To fit the hat, cover the top of your hair, pull it down on the front, then tilt to the right.

Faces never have a "perfect" balance of features, so the tilt adds a graceful balance.

Something else to bear in mind, is "hat hair." When you wear a hat, your head is warm, and sometimes a little moist, which relaxes your hair styling.

In the early twentieth century, hat fashion took account of hair fashions. So when you adopted the latest hair craze, you could easily find a hat to accommodate it.

If you want to avoid restyling your hair when you take your hat off, do something that leaves your head flat. Or copy the old-timers and leave your hat on all day.

7. Body

Select your hat in relation to the size and shape of your body, your head and height.

The goal is to ensure your head doesn't seem too big or small for your body, usually through hats that slim or widen the fullest part of your face.

For example, a large hat with a dropping brim widens your face, whereas a hat that's off your face thins and lengthens it.

A hat with a veil can soften contours, add width or height depending on their arrangement.

A large body will seem larger with a large flat-brimmed hat. If you'd like to appear smaller, try something medium to balance your head with your shoulders.

Tall, slender ladies might prefer not to wear small high hats that emphasise their slenderness.

If you're on the shorter side, you'll probably prefer a proportionally smaller hat with a smaller brim. The right trim and fabrics can appear to increase your height, without making you look like a hat stand.

It's hard to find ready-made hats in smaller sizes, so you may need to have something made to fit. You could pad the crown and sweat strap for a snug fit, but this does nothing for the problems of scale and balance.

Conversely, a tall woman in a tall hat will seem even taller, If you're self-conscious about your height, you might prefer a wider brim to balance your height. Or, depending on your facial features, a drooping brim.

And of course, if you gain or lose a lot of weight, your proportions will change, so you may need to go back to the beginning and look for a new hat.

8. Take a Long Last Look Before You Buy

If you've chosen well, your hat will become part of you. The outline of your head and hairstyle should guide the shape of it, so it frames your face and completes your outfit.

So, take a step back and look at yourself in your outfit and potential hat in a full-length mirror. Ideally from all sides to make sure it's well balanced, and you're satisfied with its appearance from all sides. Sit and stand to make sure the scale remains correct.

Look carefully to see if the colour, texture, design and trim are right for your skin tone and texture, face shape and style.

Keep trying different styles and colours to see what looks best. If you need extra time, take some photos to look at later, or ask some friends for their opinions.

Notes on Fit

I probably don't need to say it, but don't buy a hat that doesn't fit correctly because it won't feel comfortable, and you'll be worried about losing it.

A hat that fits will be snug, but not so snug it digs in.

To take your measurement, hold the tape horizontally around the circumference of your head; across your eyebrows and above your ears.

You can take it in inches or centimetres; a specialist hat shop will know what you mean.

It doesn't matter whether you wear the hat at a slant or horizontally, it will be made to fit that measurement.

Storing and Handling Your Hat

Wash your hands before handling your hat, and use both of them to minimise stretching and marking the hat (cleaning can reduce its life).

Slip a hand under the crown to lift it rather than holding the brim. When you pack it away, rest it on rolls of tissue paper to absorb any dampness, and support the shape.

Straight brim hats can rest on a flat surface, but shaped brims should hang over an edge to preserve the shape. Hats with angled brims, (e.g., trilbies) should rest upside down to protect their brims.

Straw hats are delicate and should be handled by the brims or from the insides (not by their crowns which can crack as skin oils dry out the straw). The brims are easier to clean and less likely to crack.

Care and Maintenance

Brush your hat to clean it, generally in the direction of the pile or weave. If the trim starts coming lose, stitch or glue it back into place. Alternatively, remove all the trim and clean it properly before replacing the trim.

- **Felt:** clean frequently, and don't let them get really dirty. Dip a soft cloth in cleaning solution and rub it over the felt in the direction of the nap and brush dry. Use art gum for non-liquid stains.
- **Straw:** Generally best to clean once every ten wears. Brush the dust off and redye or lacquer. If you're brave, or your hat isn't worth much, wash with soap suds (not the water) then wipe with a wet cloth and then a dry. Stuff with paper or cloth, cover with a cloth and gently iron. If necessary, reshape with your hands while damp and coat in shellac. If you need to bleach it, use a weak solution, rinse and dry in the sun.
- **Milan:** (a type of straw often dyed.) Can be cleaned with a cloth the same colour dipped in ammonia. Undyed Milan can be cleaned by dipping a cut lemon into

sulphur powder and rubbing it over the hat. Cover the whole hat in lemon sulphur and leave it to dry for an hour before brushing it off.
- **Panama:** another kind of straw, cut the end off a day-old loaf of rye bread and rub the cut end over the hat to remove the dust, then brush the bread off.
- **Velvet:** clean with solvent, brush thoroughly and remove all threads. Hold it over a steaming kettle and brush against the pile. To panne (smooth) the velvet, iron slowly in the direction of the pile. To brocade (crease) the velvet, turn it inside out with the pile inside, and twist the ends in opposite directions and leave it to dry twisted.

SUMMARY

Choosing a hat can be daunting, but there are ways to make it easier.
- Use your hat's purpose to decide how much you'll spend.
- Buy it as part of an outfit, taking colour and texture into ac-count.
- Consider the size of your body, and any facial features you might want to disguise.
- Think about it as a backdrop to your face and fair.
- Take your interest in caring for it into account.

CHAPTER 20

Clothing Care

T he most basic part of caring for your clothing is treating them well.

Before you dress in the morning, make sure your deodorants, lotions and perfumes are fully dry so that the chemicals don't damage your clothing. And if you have jewellery that might catch on your clothes, dab a little clear nail polish on the rough edges. A scarf will protect your jacket from makeup.

When you get home, make changing into your house clothes the first thing you do. Then empty your pockets, inspect your street clothes carefully and brush (stiff for dirt and dust or the Velcro kind for fibres and lint), mend or press as required before hanging them on a proper hanger that will maintain the garment's shape (not a wire one). Take the same care of your shoes and bags - inspect, wipe clean and store your shoes with shoe trees and your bags in cotton covers. De-pilling your sweaters as you go is much less tedious than taking hours to do it later. Or if you find daily is too much effort, at the very least review your clothes once a week. Maybe have a glass of wine while you do it.

Ideally you would hang them somewhere with good airflow for freshness, and leave at least 24 hours before using them again to give them a chance to relax back into their shapes. In the early twentieth century, this was outside, or on a rack fixed to a window frame to catch the breeze. Hang pants from the waist to prevent knee creasing, and belts from the buckle to prevent cracking.

This will extend the life of your clothes, and ensure that they are always fresh, wrinkle free and ready for wearing. Even if you bought them cheaply, treating them this way will extend their lives, and prepare you for taking good care of more expensive ones.

I expect that our early twentieth century counterparts would have been more tolerant of body odours than we are today, so if you are concerned by their aroma just put your clothes straight into the washing pile.

Make sure you have an appropriate moth and other insect deterrent like cedar blocks, lavender sachets or Savon de Marseille in your main clothing storage areas.

When you consider the 1900 six tub wash it's easy to see why people were interested in minimising their washing load. In fact, the traditional men's undershirt was invented to be washed more frequently than his over shirt so wear appropriate underwear like dress shields, camisoles, slips and petticoats to protect your clothes from perspiration and body oils. And use appropriate outer items like aprons and table napkins to protect your clothes from spills and splatters.

Spot cleaning becomes more difficult the longer the spot sits untreated, so flush with COOL water as soon as you become aware of a stain. Water doesn't actually work for everything, but it may prevent the stain from setting. If you know what the appropriate stain remover is and have it with you, use that instead. Do not apply heat and do not apply pressure as these can set the stain. You might want to do some research and keep a small stock of removers for the stains you commonly get.

Often the easiest thing to do is to take the garment to a dry cleaner and let them deal with it because most stains are a combination. For example, with tomato sauce you have to remove oil *and* colour. In general, you would treat one element of a stain (the oil), then wash and treat the second element (the colour), then wash and see what else needs doing.

Repairs

It's a good idea to keep a little sewing kit handy so that you can sew buttons back on before you lose them. You should have needles, thread to match the key pieces in your wardrobe, spare buttons, and safety pins.

Serious tears can be repaired invisibly by skilled tailors/dressmakers and some dry cleaners (check your phone book or app). This technique involves drawing fabric threads from the seam allowance and using them to weave the tear closed. It is very time-consuming and thus expensive, so probably only a treatment for extra special clothing.

You can prevent some tears by reinforcing the last buttons on dresses and shirts.

Fabric Care

Light colours collect dirt more quickly than dark, and soft textured faster than firm and smooth. Long fibres shed dirt more quickly than short. And when I say dirt, I also mean perspiration and body oils, makeup, food spills and so on.

Silk and most artificial silks (rayon and acetate): can be aired and pressed between wears. Iron with a low to moderate heat on the wrong side protected by a cloth or unglazed paper. Silk can be hand washed, but dry cleaning may better preserve the finish. Stained silk should definitely be dry cleaned as home spot removal can leave patches that are too clean. Dry cleaning rayon usually produces a better result than home laundering.

Wool: If you generally take good care of your wool clothing, wear appropriate under and protective clothes you can minimise the frequency and cost of cleaning. It starts with frequent airing to remove odours. Woven wool clothing should always be hung on a padded hanger to prevent the shoulders stretching, and if not being worn for some time, store them in a cotton or bamboo garment bag for protection. Knitted sweaters should be folded into drawers.

Wool absorbs moisture so it may be necessary to iron the clothes more frequently in humid climates. Gently iron from the wrong side, and protect the fabric from the heat with a damp cloth or paper. Or on a low steam setting with dry cloth/paper.

Wool knits can be hand washed, but measure the garment first (front, back and sleeve lengths, the width of back, bust and arm, front and back hip and waist) to ensure it can be stretched back to those measurements. Leave to dry flat on a towel, stretched to its original dimensions - you can carefully pin it down to ensure it doesn't shrink as it dries.

Woven wool fabrics can also be hand washed, but as many have synthetic linings it will be easiest to take these clothes to a dry cleaner.

Cotton: generally machine washable and can be hung to dry outside. Better results are obtained when colours are washed separately though you can now buy "colour catcher" sheets that absorb colour runs. Use a clean, hot (but not too hot) iron on the damp clothes on a clean smooth board.

Linen: similar to cotton, only better with a less vigorous spin to avoid deep creasing. Iron on the wrong side. The more it is washed and worn, the softer and less creased it becomes so that after a time it becomes possible to merely carefully hang clothes to dry.

Colour Care

Wash coloured clothes separately to ensure there is no colour transfer. When you hang clothes outside to dry, hang them in the shade to prevent fading. In some cases, dry cleaning can fix colours more securely to the clothing fibres.

Dry Cleaning

Dry cleaning uses toxic and dangerous chemicals and is best dealt with by professionals. Good dry cleaning can prolong the life of your clothes. If you have precious buttons, you should cover them with foil for protection. It's worth mentioning that there are shoulder pads as well, just to make sure they stay put.

When you take in stained clothes, tell the cleaner where the stains are located and what they are from to ensure their proper treatment.

Many dry cleaners also offer small repair and alteration services. These are convenient, but they can also be expensive.

When you get your clothes home, take them out of the plastic and air them outside to allow the chemicals to dissipate before placing on proper solid and supportive hangers in your closet. Or in a cotton or bamboo garment bag if you won't be wearing them for a time.

Make sure that your monthly budget includes a sum for proper cleaning as required.

Hand Washing

Start by cleaning and rinsing the sink or basin you plan to use, and then half fill with lukewarm or tepid water somewhere in the 86 - 104° F (30 - 40° C) range). Add a few drops of a mild detergent - look for one labelled delicate and/or woollens.

Put your garment in and swish it around in the water, gently scrunching or kneading a few times. The goal is just to push the water through the weave so that it will take light soil as it goes. Remove the garment from the wash water and gently compress to remove excess water. Wash each garment individually; if they are not too dirty you can use the same water.

Then rinse each item and squeeze out the water. You can roll it up in a towel to start the drying process, but the best results for maintaining its shape are achieved by laying it flat.

Some garment labels permit machine washing on a gentle or delicate cycle, and this may be preferable for larger, sturdier clothes like cotton knits and some spandex sportswear. You could use a lingerie bag for additional protection for less sturdy clothes.

Ironing

Choose an iron that offers a good shot of steam, and a board that is well padded. Metallic covers reflect the heat back onto the garment and this can damage delicate fabrics; plain cotton covers provide better protection. Your pressing cloth should be a good quality plain cotton, preferably not dyed or bleached. If you are serious about your ironing you might also like a sleeve board, seam roll (so you don't get seam allowance creases), pressing mitt (for hard to reach areas) and/or a sole plate cover to protect delicate and synthetic items. Many modern irons are self-cleaning, but if you don't have one of those get some iron cleaner to ensure the sole is clean and flat when you come to use it.

Start by making sure the iron is not too hot - test on an inconspicuous area. If you don't have a sole plate, iron on the wrong side. Iron the part of the garment that is least likely to crease first (for example, the collar), then those more likely to wrinkle (sleeves and body). If you like crisp creases, leave the garment to cool on the board because they may fall out if you leave them to cool on a hanger. You could also use a little spray starch for crispness.

Freezing

If your clothes or shoes are not badly soiled (or smelly), you can place them in the freezer to kill bugs and germs. This is particularly popular for ensuring jeans don't lose their comfortable lived in feeling. It can help control sneaker odour as well. Just make sure you put them in a bag before they go in the freezer to protect both your clothes and your food.

Shoes

At the end of the day inspect and wipe clean your shoes. Store them with shoe trees to ensure they keep their shape and are adequately aired. Leave for at least 24 hours to allow the perspiration to evaporate before wearing them again. If possible, apply some shoe polish to nourish the leather but don't forget to wipe them clean before you wear them again!

Suede shoes often lose colour at the toes very quickly, and if they are not a common colour you should take them to a cobbler to see if they can be recoloured (you may be able to do black and dark brown yourself).

When the soles of your favourite shoes are worn, take them to the cobbler to have them resoled and/or reheeled.

If you buy leather soled shoes have them soled and heeled before you wear them. The leather sole is not as durable as modern polymers, and will not repel water when the ground is wet. In the early twentieth century you would buy goloshes, to wear over your shoes to protect them from the wet weather - they are still available but harder to come by.

SUMMARY

Cleaning and mending your clothes, shoes and other accessories promptly and properly will maximise their useful lives. Airing them out between wears and storing them correctly will ensure they are always ready to wear.

CHAPTER 21

Maintaining Your Body

If you'are hoping to make a long-term wardrobe plan, we now need to deal with the rather large elephant in the room. Your long term plan assumes that your body shape is more or less stable and that you can rely on it having more or less the same dimensions for the three to five year span of your plan. This means you need to take charge of yourself and in the same way that you have made some basic decisions about how you are going to dress your body, you need to make some more about how you are going to treat it.

Like the rest of this book, this information comes from the early twentieth century; I have taken interesting and still relevant information and compiled it into general principles for living. It is offered for entertainment and inspiration, not as serious and reliable advice. If you have not recently lived the healthiest life, seek medical advice before you make any changes, particularly if you are managing medical conditions.

Leaving your clothing choices out of it, your authentic beauty is made up of five elements; your body, posture, carriage, facial features and complexion. Looking your most beautiful requires that you make the best of these elements, and this means you need to maintain good health.

Your most important beauty tool is weight control through diet and exercise. Others are skin care, dealing with stress, sleeping well and maintaining your hair, eyes and teeth. Your goal should be to perfect healthy living because neglect in one element drags the others down.

Body

For a nicely curved feminine figure, you need a good balance of lean muscle and fat. Too much fat is ugly and unhealthy, it is not your natural state to be fat. Fat people are generally not physically strong, and you need to be strong to keep your body and mind beautiful and efficient. When you are strong, your muscles (and shape) are in the places you need and want them for good posture and carriage; your arms, legs and chest.

If you aren't sure whether you need to lose weight, here are some handy indicators from 1918 that you do: rolls of loose flesh, loose fleshy abdomen, loose bust, excessive hips, puffy knees and ankles.

Posture

Good posture is where you think, stand and walk tall; up straight and not slouching. You might imagine that you are a building four stories tall - feet, hips, chest and head, all balanced securely upon each other, and that the elevator descending from your ear will pass through the middle of your shoulder, hip, knee and ankle. Or that you have a weight passing vertically through your body from head to pelvis that prevents you from leaning too far forward or backwards.

CARRIAGE

Carriage is your posture in motion. Good posture contributes to a smooth, fluid, graceful and efficient walk, and walking develops the muscular strength and suppleness that results in good posture. Balance your weight on the balls of your feet, walking briskly in evenly spaced steps.

When your carriage is good, the organs sit in their proper places where they can carry out their work unimpeded. Bad carriage leads to muscle and ligature strain, dislocation and compression of internal organs, and dislocations of the spine. Straightening out the kinks in your spine can add as much as an inch (2.5 cm) to your height along with all the health benefits that come from uncompressing your organs. Stretching benefits the nervous systems and opens up space for blood to flow as well as going some way to correcting slouching.

When women wear heels, they throw their weight forward onto their toes, and this puts a strain on the whole body and causes backaches. This can be helped with back exercises and moderate height heels.

Graceful movement is a matter of confidence and self-expression. The confidence comes from well-practised control of your movement; initially it takes constant effort and monitoring, but over time becomes automatic.

FACE

While your genes give you your basic face shape and structure, good health gives you the good muscle tone (fewer wrinkles) and clear fresh complexion (less acne) that expresses your combination of beauty and soul. Good diet, exercise, adequate sleep and plenty of water are all essential for good skin.

To control acne and remove blackheads, use a soft complexion brush and soapy water in the evening and rinse with warm then cool water. Don't squeeze them; they return quickly and you risk scarring and infection. Pimples and rough skin on the back can be removed with a firm brush and soapy water - dry skin thoroughly.

To dispel existing wrinkles and prevent new ones, cultivate a calm face; teach yourself not to let fleeting emotions chase across it, and don't allow yourself to frown. During your daily cleanse and moisturise give yourself a firm light face and neck massage to get your blood moving and relax your facial muscles and/or get regular facials.

Eyes

Dull eyes with dark bags are caused by bad diet and lack of exercise - lack of sleep doesn't help either. Most of us use at least two kinds of computing equipment almost non-stop all day long. Reset your eyes periodically by looking up from close work and into the distance, then exercise your muscles by rolling your eyes. You can stimulate blood flow by gently tapping closed eyes and correct visual deficiencies with glasses.

Teeth

White teeth and fresh breath are assets. Clean your teeth and rinse with antiseptic mouthwash morning and night. Visit a dentist for a professional clean twice a year.

Hair

Glossy, thick, beautiful hair will enhance your face while bad hair will detract. Healthy hair grows as much as 1" (2.5 cm) per month, unhealthy hair much less. Aside from good diet and exercise, glorious hair only requires five minutes morning and night brushing to maintain condition (50 smooth strokes with a stiff bristle brush). Brushing removes dust, distributes oil (which makes hair shiny) and stimulates the scalp.

If you do not use a lot of hair product or processing, you probably won't need to shampoo more than once a fortnight (maybe a little more or less depending on its oiliness and general condition) with a pure soap (e.g. shaving soap) and soft water (clean rain water is best). Wash your brushes weekly.

Hands

Soft smooth hands suggest beauty and efficiency. Protect your hands with gloves where possible (with practice you will become quite dexterous). Renew them with lotion, massaging in well before bed and sleeping in a pair of gloves. If your hands are stained, bleach them with a lemon juice rinse. Ugly nails make ugly hands, so give yourself a manicure once a week, and rub a little hand cream into your nails each day.

Feet

Your feet are quite technical, with 26 bones held together by ligaments and muscles. If they are not treated well and securely housed in well-fitted shoes, they will not work together properly; you will have with blisters and very sore feet. The bulk of your body weight is supported by the arch of your foot, and wearing heels that are too high or not well placed will unbalance your load carrying capacity by forcing your weight onto your toes with your back, neck and legs taking up the strain of keeping your body in balance. Wider heels give better support, and are more suitable for everyday activities.

Strong healthy feet are beautiful, and as they don't hurt, are good for a wrinkle free face as well! Good shoes that adequately support the arch are essential for this, and for graceful movement with smooth carriage. Do not wear old shoes with rundown or turned over heels. Good shoes will prevent further damage, but you may still need to deal with the effects of previous abuse such as corns and bunions. Use a pumice stone to remove rough skin and cut your nails carefully.

Change your shoes frequently; allow at least a day for the perspiration to dry out between wears. Bathe your feet gently and massage with vinegar or alcohol to prevent perspiration.

DIET

You are lucky enough live in a time where good quality fresh produce is abundant. It is so abundant that you probably throw away more than you eat. You might think that you don't have the time to prepare nutritious food, but you can have a healthy and delicious meal on the table ready to eat within thirty minutes of walking in your door. If you don't know how, type "quick and healthy meals" into your favourite search engine and see what comes up. Or treat yourself to a cooking class.

Do not eat if you're not hungry. A grumbly tummy does not necessarily mean you are hungry - it could just be the expectation of food or some other disorder of the digestion such as constipation.

When you eat, choose food that supplies nutrients without adding to your fat load, and eat in moderation. Don't restrict any foods, but select simple foods like vegetables to ensure sufficient fibre, minerals, vitamins and organic acids for preference. Train yourself to prefer fruits that don't require additional sweetness and simple desserts over pastries, greasy food, sugar, candies and heavy puddings.

Chew thoroughly and leave the table with the capacity to eat more. Drink plenty of water between meals. Change your cooking methods to limit the amount of added fat.

EXERCISE

Our bodies developed to support a life where vigorous activity was essential for existence. Inactive bodies do not generate good blood flow. Well-chosen energetic exercises will move most of the larger muscles. Even just standing rather than sitting uses 40% more energy. Walking more than 100% over standing, running three times more and swimming four times.

Expending energy in this way consumes oxygen from the air and nutrients from food, combining them to make pure blood. A few minutes two or three times a day keeps the whole body stimulated, with the internal fat burning activity continuing when the external ceases.

Walking is the easiest exercise to get started with, and in 1918 the recommendation was a mere 75 minutes daily before breakfast (yes, an hour and a quarter). Most of us would say that's just feasible with all the other things we think we have to do.

Elite athletes are advised to eat two to four hours before exercise so if you can only do a quick stroll around the block to start with, do it before breakfast. Exercise also changes your blood chemistry and suppresses your appetite for a time, so while you will eat less breakfast, you will be hungrier later and may need to be careful not to eat more energy than you use.

Outdoor swimming combines the benefits of exercise, the invigoration of a cold plunge bath with fresh air and sunshine. It requires good control of muscles and delivers poise which is the basis of beauty, dignity and confidence. It also benefits complexion, stimulates organs and develops muscles.

Dancing exercises both mind and body and develops grace and good health. Take a class or put some music on and use your whole body to freely express the mood of it. Dance like no one is watching!

Managing Stress

Stress is the cause of many bad lifestyle choices. You can minimise stress by balancing your work and play; allowing a couple of hours to maintain your physical wellbeing and not devoting all of your spare time to caring for your family. Make time to enjoy music, reading and the theatre. If you entertain at night, consider napping or relaxing during the day, but not too much because that is just lazy.

Knowing how you feel when you are stressed can help you identify your stress triggers and understand when you need to manage them. Knowing what relaxes you will help you manage stress, and prevent it from building up.

If you are having trouble sleeping, take exercise, avoid mental stimulation in the evening and go to bed early. Have a warm bath, drink some warm milk, eat a light dinner, and go to bed expecting to sleep.

Summary

Authentic beauty comes from a shapely body, good posture, smooth carriage, a relaxed face and clear complexion; these are only achievable through good health.

You can support your good health and beauty through diet, exercise, sleep and stress management. Maintaining a suitable skin care routine and taking care of your hair, eyes and teeth are important too.

Glossary

A-line: a skirt that is fitted at the hip and widens toward the hem like the letter A.

AC (Alternating Current): developed by Nikola Tesla, alternating current is now the principal form of household electrical supply because it is easy to change the voltage. It occurs when the charge carriers periodically reverse direction, and can vary in magnitude. For example, in the US it is supplied at 60 hertz (60 reversals per second) and in the UK 50.

Accessory: an additional item to complete an outfit such as shoes, bag, jewellery, gloves, belt and so on.

Acetate: a fibre manufactured from cotton or wood. It looks shiny and is commonly used in eveningwear.

Acrylic: a synthetic fibre with a wool-like feel that can be manufactured in a variety of weights and feels. It is commonly used as a wool replacement, but is also used in faux fur.

Appropriate: A garment is appropriate if it is suitable for the activities you undertake, in the places that you usually find yourself doing them.

Average: a quantity that represents the typical. It is calculated by adding all the results and dividing the sum by the number of results.

Babydoll: originally a short, high-waisted loose sleeveless nightgown, now available as a daywear dress.

Balloon Jacket: a short spherical jacket. Sometimes worn with a spherical balloon skirt.

Bias Cut: the fabric is cut diagonally rather than straight. It results in a slightly clingy garment with a more fluid drape.

Brim: the bottom part of the hat that protrudes from the crown and shades the face.

BTU: British Thermal Units. One BTU is the amount of work required to raise the temperature of one pound (454 g) of water by 1°F (0.56°C). In terms of power (as used in the book) it is about 0.3 of a Watt. It can also be expressed in terms of energy at 253 calories (1.06 kilojoules).

Budget: an amount of money assigned for a specified purpose, in this case, for clothing.

Camisole: originally a dainty corset cover, with a straight top and ribbon shoulder straps, now used as a slip or to add a layer for warmth.

Capsule: the basis of your wardrobe - a small core collection of good quality clothing, supplemented by "extras", that meets your daily needs for four or five years. See also cluster and minimalist.

Carriage: your bearing; the way you hold and move your head and body.

Chemise Dress: originally a knee-length sleeveless straight cut unfitted undergarment that hung from the shoulders and combined the functions of corset cover and short petticoat, now worn as a dress.

Cinderella Clothes: your everyday clothes.

Closet: the place where you store all your clothes whether this is a cupboard, chest of drawers, a room or all of them.

Clothing Forms: forms such as dress, pant, skirt, and top.

Cluster: a small set of themed clothes such as summer holidays, work or eveningwear. See also capsule and minimalist wardrobe.

Cocoon Coat: a loose draped coat, more recently called a Big Coat or Man's Coat.

Column Dress: a long sleeveless, narrow fitted dress that is often beaded, embroidered or otherwise embellished.

Corsage: once a dress's waist or bodice, now used to describe a bunch of flowers pinned on the waist or shoulder.

Corset or Corsets: a close-fitting undergarment enclosing the trunk, stiffened with whalebone or similar material and capable of being tightened by lacing. Also known as stays.

Cold Cream: an emulsion of water and fat used for removing makeup, moisturising and as a shaving cream.

Cost per Wear: the amount of money each wear of an item costs. Calculated by dividing the purchase price (plus in some cases maintenance cost), by the number of wears.

Couturier: a dress designer based in France. This is the masculine version and the feminine is couturière, though this form is no longer common.

Cowl: a draped fold of fabric at the front (neck) or back (drape) of a garment.

Crown: the top of a hat. The crown may be shaped with a crease on the insde, and dents on the outside. (You'll often see people handling the hat with these in old movies.)

Daywear: clothes to wear during the day, generally made of plain cotton or wool fabrics that provide greater body coverage with high necklines and long sleeves.

DC (Direct Current): now only available in batteries. In this form of current, the charge flows in one direction with very little variation in magnitude.

Drapery: loose garments that hang in folds.

Draping: a form of dressmaking where fabric is positioned and pinned on a dress form and then used as a pattern to construct the final garment.

Dress Clips: a clip attached to a dress to highlight an attractive feature such as the neckline or a lapel. They came in similar styles and materials to brooches.

Dressmaker: a person who makes and alters women's clothing.

Dress Shields: pads basted (tacked) into a dress' armpits to absorb perspiration and prevent it reaching the garment. In the early twentieth-century, they were removed and washed separately, but you can buy disposable adhesive ones now.

Earth Closet: Over time there have been several variations of this form of toilet. At its most basic it was a small shed in the garden containing a seat with a hole in it and a bucket underneath to catch the excrement. Private closets would be manually emptied by the owner into a composting system or burned, whereas public would be emptied by the municipal authority. Alternatively, the shed was built over a deep hole in the ground into which a shovel of dirt would be emptied on the top to reduce the smell and insect problem. Both these systems were also used for kitchen and household waste.

Empire: a short waisted dress with short full sleeves and long loose skirt. Now more commonly refers to any garment with a waistline that falls just below the bust.

Eveningwear: clothes for evening events, generally made of luxurious and embellished fabrics that provide less body coverage with low necklines and short sleeves.

Everyday Clothes: clothes worn frequently in ordinary daily life.

Fabric: cloth made from yarns that are woven, knitted or bonded.

Fibre: the raw material that is spun into yarns and then knitted, woven or fused to become fabric. May come from animal, vegetable and mineral sources.

Fitted: a garment that loosely follows the body's contours.

Gaiters: ankle coverings made of cloth or leather that zip or button up the side and are secured by a strap that runs under the foot.

Godet: a shaped section of a woman's skirt that is wider at the bottom than at the top to add fullness at the hem.

Goloshes (Galoshes): waterproof overshoes, particularly for high heels. Also known as rubbers and overshoes.

Good Clothes: generally higher quality clothes worn less frequently at particular times when you want to look your best such as church, events and occasions.

Halterneck: a strap that runs from the front of a garment, round the back of the neck to the other side. They are generally sleeveless and leave the back uncovered.

Haute Couture: handmade high-end made-to-measure fashion made from high quality fabrics and finishes. The term originally referred to clothes made by the House of Worth in Paris, expanded to French fashion houses, but is now a protected term with restricted use.

High Waisted: the waist of the garment sits higher than your natural waist. See also low waisted.

Hobble Dress: a dress with a narrow hem that restricts the stride. Some had tight restrictive skirts, others external trim that gathered in the fullness. Also skirts.

House Clothes: clothes worn in private.

Icebox: an insulated cupboard with a compartment to contain a large block of ice used to cool or preserve food and drinks.

Jersey: a stretchy knit fabric used in clothing like t-shirts. It can be made from silk, wool, cotton or linen as well as synthetic fibres and blends. It comes in a variety of weights and stretches.

Kellermanns: a fitted thigh length one piece swimsuit with a fitted knee length skirt worn over the top for modesty.

Leg Break: the place where your leg meets your body, just above the thigh. It bends when you lift your leg.

Leisurewear: informal, comfortable clothing designed for resting or relaxing. Usually a form of house clothing.

Lifestyle Categories: the groups your life falls into, like career and leisure.

Low Waisted: the waist of the garment sits lower than your natural waist. Also known as drop waist. See also high waisted.

Made-to-Measure: clothing that is constructed to a customer's body measurements rather than a "standard" size.

Magazine Spread Technique: a technique for learning to see yourself as a whole rather than body parts. Take a lot of photos of yourself and print them (several to a page). Look at them as if they are a magazine spread featuring a designer's new collection.

Manufactured Fibres: (also known as man-made fibres) these fibres are altered from their natural state in a manufacturing process where they may be dissolved and treated before a thread is drawn out. Common fibres include rayon and acetate. See also natural and synthetic fibres.

Mary Janes: these shoes have a low heel, rounded toe box and are fastened by a strap across the foot. This style has been worn by both sexes for hundreds of years throughout the world. They take their current name from a character in the comic strip *Buster Brown* as a result of a licensing deal between the cartoonist Richard Felton Outcault and the Brown Shoe Company in 1904.

Median: the middle number of a sequence, representing the centre of a distribution.

Minimalist Wardrobe: a small number of clothes that comprise your entire wardrobe. See also capsule and cluster.

Modacrylic: a synthetic fibre similar to acrylic though flame retardant.

Mousseline (de soie): a transparent but firm silk material with an even weave. Similar to chiffon, gauze or tulle.

Natural Fibres: naturally occurring fibres that are not significantly changed by the manufacturing process which mainly consists of cleaning and spinning. Common fibres include animal (wool, mohair, silk), vegetable (cotton, hemp, flax, linen) and mineral (asbestos). See also manufactured and synthetic fibres.

Nylon: a strong and durable synthetic fibre with useful wash and wear properties. It is soft to the touch and recovers well from stretching.

Outfit: all the clothes and accessories that complete a look. May include a dress, hat, shoes, hosiery, gloves, handkerchief, handbag, jewellery, umbrella, coat and underwear.

Pencil Skirt: a modern form of hobble skirt. It is slim fitted with a narrow straight cut. Some have a split or pleat to provide ease of movement.

Personality Type One: a person that retains their youthful outlook and manner their whole life and consequently choose simple clothing in bright colours, busy patterns and fluffy designs. The "girl next door" easy going and comfort driven dresser.

Personality Type Two: has a delicate soft appearance and prefers soft flowing fabrics, pastel shades in loose full styles.

Personality Type Three: is understated and elegant, prefers balance and symmetry. Likes draped clothes in dark subdued colours and richly textured fabrics.

Personality Type Four: actively participates in business and sport, may appear to have severely tailored features. They prefer plain clothes made from stiff fabrics with severe lines which can produce a striking, head-turning look.

Petite Fit: a range of clothing designed for women who are 5' 3" (160 cm) or 5' 4" (162 cm) or less (brand dependent). These garments have shorter sleeve, leg, and body lengths to produce a proportional fit, as well as scaled placement of darts, buttons and trims. If they are properly scaled, they will fit better and alterations will be less obvious than regular fit garments. See also regular and tall fits.

Petticoat: originally a short jacket worn by men under a longer coat, becoming a woman's decorated shirt under an open gown and then an underskirt.

Pleat (Plait): a type of trim where fabric is folded in on itself. It comes in several varieties; accordion, box, cartridge, kilt, knife, and sunburst.

Polyamide: can be a natural fibre in the form of silk and wool, but more commonly understood as a synthetic, generally sold as nylon.

Polyester: a synthetic fibre that is strong and durable, resistant to wrinkles, moulds, most chemicals and friction. It is also resistant to water and thus quick drying. It retains its shape well.

Posture: the position of the body and the position of its limbs. Generally, good posture results when the spine is aligned and the joints are not bent.

Princess Clothes: your good clothes, particularly the ones you will probably never wear.

Purchasing Principles: a series of choices about what is appropriate and stylish to guide your shopping. They include things like fabrics and colours, quality and practicality that manifest in general decisions like buying only natural fibres, skirts without pockets or stiletto heels.

Quality: a good quality garment is one that fulfils the requirements of its form and function, for example, a sweater that looks good and keeps you warm.

Rayon: fibres manufactured from cotton or wood derived cellulose and woven into a wide range of fabrics including crepe, satin and taffeta.

Ready-to-Wear: factory made clothing in a range of standardised sizes sold as finished garments that can be worn as is.

Regular Fit: these are the so-called standard sizes designed for statistically average women who are 5'5" - 5' 9" (163 - 175 cm) tall. See also petite and tall fits.

Rouge: also known as blush - can be powder or cream.

Ruching: a process of pleating, gathering or ruffling fabric. It can be added as a trim, or inserted into a garment as a decorative element.

Sack Dress: like a chemise dress (straight cut unfitted dress that hangs from the shoulders) but with sleeves and available in longer and shorter lengths.

Semifitted: a garment that loosely follows the body's contours.

Sheath Dress: similar to a column dress (a narrow fitted dress) but knee length and unembellished.

Shift Dress: the same as a sack dress (loose dress without belt that hangs straight from the shoulders) only sounds nicer and is therefore more popular.

Shirtwaist: precursor to the modern blouse, and as the Garibaldi shirt, the first separate garment for women. Also describes a women's tailored blouse or shirt, and the sort of dress that is essentially a long shirt.

Shopping Principles: a series of commitments that reduce stress and help you to make good buying decisions. These include things like sticking to your plan, buying only amazing clothes, being nice to sales assistants and stopping when it gets too much.

Signature: something that identifies a person and sets them apart from others.

Slip: a detachable dress lining. Originally made and sold with the dress, but more recently an independent undergarment worn with many dresses.

Sportswear: originally a term for clothing worn during sporting activities, but by the 1920s and 30s had broadened to include watching sport and is now commonly used to describe a uniquely American style of casual dress.

Staples: things like socks and underwear you can't do without.

Street Clothes: clothes worn in public.

Style: A person's individual expression of their personality through the colour and shape of their clothing choices.

Synthetic Fibres: Made from chemicals, generally by-products of petroleum processing. Common fibres include nylon, acrylic, polyurethane, and polypropylene. See also manufactured and natural fibres.

Tailor: a person who makes or alters clothes, particularly menswear in the form of suits, coats, and other outer garments.

Tailored: a plain garment with simple straight lines OR a garment that has been altered to fit better by a tailor (or these days a dressmaker).

Tall Fit: a range of clothing designed for women who are 5' 9" (175 cm) or 5' 10" (178 cm) or taller. These garments have longer sleeve, leg, and body lengths to produce a proportional fit, as well as scaled placement of darts, buttons and trims. If they are properly scaled, they will fit better and alterations will be less obvious than regular fit garments. See also petite and regular fits.

Ten Item Wardrobe: a collection of ten core items of clothing supplemented by extras. The core items will generally be your middle layers (e.g. dresses, jeans, tops) supplemented by extras; your under and outer layers and accessories.

Thermoplastic: a plastic that is soft and pliable when heated with no loss of characteristics. They can be heated and cooled as many times as necessary to achieve the desired end result.

Thermoset: plastics that retain their strength and shape when heated and cannot be remoulded.

Trim: the hat's decoration, commonly a hatband made of ribbon. Sometimes tied in a bow, some-times beads, buttons, feathers and flowers at-tached to the band. In some hats the brim may be bound as well.

Tunic: originally an undergarment worn by Ancient Roman soldiers, and later a long sleeved knee length Saxon outer garment with side splits from the hip. May be fitted or gathered at the waist.

Viscose: a form of rayon that is semi-synthetic fibre derived from regenerated cellulose.

Wardrobe: all your clothes.

Wardrobe Plan: your programme for buying clothes that you can afford, are appropriate for your life and meet your style needs.

Warp: The warp threads are the long threads attached to the loom. They are generally worn vertically on your body.

Wasp Waist: an extreme form of the hourglass figure where the waist is compressed by corsetry to produce a sharp break between the natural rib in to a small waist and out to hips as seen in a wasp's segmented body. This waist measured 16" - 18" (41.64 - 45.72 cm) against a more usual measurement of 20" - 23" (50.8 - 58.42 cm).

Weft: The weft threads are woven crosswise back and forth through the warp to form the fabric. They are generally worn horizontally across the body. Also known as woof.

Wellingtons: waterproof boots; traditionally mid-calf but available ranging from ankle to knee height. Also known as gum or rain boots.

Wrap Dress: a dress that closes at the front when one side is fastened over the other side. This fastening forms a V neck. The dresses can be fitted or straight. Also available in a faux version that does not open in the front and in skirts

Yarns: fibres spun together to create thicker, stronger and more flexible threads.

Yoke: the part of a dress that is fitted to the shoulders or a skirt that is fitted to the hips from which the rest of the garment is sewn. Sometimes in gathers or pleats.

Bibliography

Abbott, Walter F. 1981. "Income Level and Inflation Strain in the United States: 1971-1975" *American Journal of Economics and Sociology* 40 (2): 97-106.

About the 301. 2014. Singer301.com. http://singer301.com/about/default.html.

Agency for Toxic Substances & Disease Registry. 2015. "Public Health Statement for Naphthalene, 1-Methylnaphthalene, and 2-Methylnaphthalene". Centers for Disease Control and Prevention. http://www.atsdr.cdc.gov/phs/phs.asp?id=238&tid=43.

Andre, Mary Lou. 2004. *Ready to Wear: An Expert's Guide to Choosing and Using Your Wardrobe*. New York: A Perigee Book.

Andrews, Benjamin R. 1920. "Thrift as a Family and Individual Problem Some Standard Budgets." *Annals of the American Academy of Political and Social Science* 87 (January): 11-20.

Baxter, Laura and Alpha Latzke. 1949. *Today's Clothing*. Chicago: J.B. Lippincott Company.

Betters, Paul Vernon. 1930. *The Bureau of Home Economics: Its History, Activities and Organization*. Washington: The Brookings Institution. http://babel.hathitrust.org/cgi/pt?id=coo.31924003540436;view=1up;seq=1.

Black, Sandy. 2006. *Fashioning Fabrics: Contemporary Textiles in Fashion*. London: Black Dog Publishing.

Brady, Dorothy S. 1951. "Scales of Living and Wage Earners' Budgets." *Annals of the American Academy of Political and Social Science* 274 (March): 32-38.

Brown, Clair. 1994. *American Standards of Living 1918-1988*. Cambridge Massachusetts: Blackwell Publishers.

Carver, Courtney. 2015. PROJECT 333: Simple Is The New Black. http://theproject333.com.

Clancy, Mary. 2007. "Working lives, women's lives: some research sources and possibilities." *Saothar* 32: 65-69.

Clouting, Laura. 2015. "10 Top Tips For Winning At 'Make Do And Mend' Imperial War Museums. https://www.iwm.org.uk/history/10-top-tips-for-winning-at-make-do-and-mend.

Cooper, Grace Rogers. 1976. *The Sewing Machine.* Washington DC: Smithsonian Institute.

Costantino, Maria. 1997. *Men's Fashion in the Twentieth Century: From Frock Coats to Intelligent fibres.* New York: Costume & Fashion Press.

Cox, Angie and Greg Cox. 2015. You Look Fab. http://youlookfab.com/.

DeWitt, John W. 1994. "Sewing machines show few advances in 160 years." *Apparel Industry Magazine* 55(9): 38-39.

Dirix, Emanuele, and Charlotte Fiell. 2013. *1940s Fashion: The Definitive Sourcebook.* London: Goodman Fiell.

Ewers, William, H.W. Baylor and H.H. Kenaga. 1970. *Sincere's History of the Sewing Machine.* Phoenix: Sincere Press.

Fallon, James. 1992. "The English Version." *Daily News Record* 22 May: 146.

Fashion Era. 2004. http://www.fashion-era.com.

Faux, Susie. 1999. *Wardrobe Solutions: A Total System for Dressing with Style and Confidence.* London: Marshall Publishing.

Fiell, Charlotte, and Emmanuelle Dirix, eds. 2011. *Fashion Sourcebook 1920s.* Fiell Publishing.

Fiell, Charlotte, and Emmanuelle Dirix, eds. 2012. *1930s Fashion: The Definitive Sourcebook.* London: Goodman Fiell Publishing.

Fox, Bonnie 1990. "Selling the Mechanized Household: 70 Years of Ads in Ladies Home Journal" *Gender and Society* 4 (1): 25-40.

Frederick, Christine. 1924. "New Wealth, New Standards of Living and Changed Family Budgets." *Annals of the American Academy of Political and Social Science.* 115 (September): 74-82.

Garcia, Nina. 2007. *The Little Black Book of Style.* New York, Collins.

Gazeley, Ian and Andrew Newell. 2010. "Poverty in Edwardian Britain" *The Economic History Review* 64 (1): 52–71.

Glamour Daze: A Vintage Fashion and Beauty Archive. 2009. http://glamourdaze.com.

Gunn, Tim with Kate Maloney. 2007. *A Guide to Quality, Taste & Style*. New York: Abrams Image.

Hawkins, John. 2013. "A sartorial tale: Evening wear for men: The style and the times" *The World of Antiques & Art* 85: 18-25.

Heisig, Jan Paul. 2011. "Who Does More Housework: Rich or Poor? A Comparison of 33 Countries." *American Sociological Review* 76 (1): 74-99.

Helmbold, Lois Rita and Ann Schofield. 1989. "Women's Labor History, 1790-1945." *Reviews in American History* 17 (4): 501-518.

Hillis, Marjorie. 1937. *Orchids on Your Budget: Or Live Smartly on What Have You*. Great Britain: Virago Press reprint 2009. ISBN: 9781844086186.

Horowitz, Daniel. 1985. "Frugality or Comfort: Middle-Class Styles of Life in the Early Twentieth Century." *American Quarterly* 37 (2): 239-259.

Imperial War Museums. 2014. "8 Facts About Clothes Rationing In Britain During The Second World War." Imperial War Museums. http://www.iwm.org.uk/history/8-facts-about-clothes-rationing-in-britain-during-the-second-world-war.

Jett, Tish. 2013. *Forever Chic: Frenchwomen's Secrets for Timeless Beauty, Style and Substance*. New York: Rizzoli ex Libras

Kellerman, Annette. 1918. *Physical Beauty: How to Keep It*. New York: George H. Dorian Company.

Latzke, Alpha and Beth Quinlan. 1935. *Clothing: An Introductory College Course*. JB Lippincott.

Lever, James. 2002. *Costume and Fashion: A Concise History*. New York: Thames & Hudson Inc. 4th ed.

Loewen, Jane. 1926. *Millinery*. New York: Macmillan Co.

McCleary, Ann. 1982. "Work in Progress: Domesticity and the Farm Woman: A Case Study of Women in Augusta County, Virginia 1850 - 1940." *Perspectives in Vernacular Architecture* 1:25-30.

MacLeod, W.M. 1961. "A Note on the 1947-8 Family Budget Survey" *The Canadian Journal of Economics and Political Science/ Revue canadienne d'Economique et de Science politique* 27 (2): 243-247.

Moshe, William E. 1921. *Minimum Quantity and Cost Budgets for Clerical Workers in New York City.* New York: Bureau of Municipal Research and Training School for Public Service.

Nix-Rice, Nancy. 1996. *Looking Good: A Comprehensive Guide to Wardrobe Planning, Color & Personal Style Development.* Portland: Palmer/Pletsch Incorporated.

Patty, Virgina. C.1925. *Hats and How to Make Them.* Seattle: Rand McNally & Company.

Palmieri, Jean E. 1999. "Royal Treatments 1900s." *Daily News Record* 14 May.

Peixotto, Jessica B. 1929. "Family Budgets of Faculty Members" *Bulletin of the American Association of University Professors* 15 (2): 144-149.

Perkin, Joan. 2002. "Sewing machines: Liberation or drudgery for women?" *History Today* 52(12): 35-41.

Phillips, Charles, Neil Grant, Margaret Mulvihill, David Gould, Trevor Morris, Mark Barrett and Reg Grant. 2000. *The 20th Century Year by Year: The People and Events That Shaped the Last Hundred Years.* London: Marshall Publishing Ltd.

Picken, Mary Books. 1918. *The Secrets of Distinctive Dress: Harmonious, becoming and beautiful dress - its value and how to achieve it.* Scranton: The Women's Institute of Domestic Arts and Sciences.

Przybyszewski, Linda. 2014. *The Lost Art of Dress: The Women Who Once Made America Stylish.* New York: Basic Books.

Reed, Ellery F. 1946. "Cost of Living Compared with Family Income in Seven Cities" *American Sociological Review* 11 (2): 192-197.

Rosen, Ellen Israel. 2002. *Making Sweatshops: The Globalization of the U.S. Apparel Industry*. Berkeley: University of California Press.

Ross, John ed. 1999. *Chronicle of the 20th Century*. Ringwood: Penguin Books Australia.

Scott, Jennifer L. 2011. *Lessons from Madame Chic: 20 Stylish Secrets I Learned While Living in Paris*. New York: Simon and Schuster.

Scott, Peter M. and James Walker. 2012. "Working-Class Household Consumption Smoothing in Interwar Britain" *The Journal of Economic History* 72 (3): 797-825.

Silver, Cameron. 2012. *Decades: One Hundred Years of Timeless Style*. London: Bloomsbury.

Smith, Patty Rai. 2004. *Building a Basic Wardrobe by Clusters*. Lexington: University of Kentucky Cooperative Extension.

Stecker, Margaret L. 1937. *Intercity differences in costs of living in March, 1935, 59 cities*. Washington: US Government Printing Office.

Strasser, Susan. 1982. *Never Done; A History of American Housework*. New York: Pantheon Books.

Taggart, Judie and Jackie Walker. 2003. *"I Don't Have a Thing to Wear": The Psychology of Your Closet*. New York: Pocket Books.

Thomas, Pauline and Guy Thomas. 2014. Fashion Era. http://www.fashion-era.com/index.htm.

Todd, Selina. 2004. "Young Women, Work and Family in Inter-War Rural England." *The Agricultural History Review*. 52 (1): 83-98.

Tortora, Phyllis G. 2015. *Dress, Fashion, and Technology: From Prehistory to the Present*. London: Bloomsbury Academic.

United States Congress. 1911. *Senate Select committee on wages and prices of commodities: Investigation relative to wages and prices of commodities*. Washington: Government Printing Office.

United States Department of Labor. 1941. *Changes in Cost of Living in Large Cities in the US 1913 - 1941: Bulletin 669*. Washington: United States Government Printing Office.

United States Department of Labor. 1942. *Handbook of Labor Statistics: Volume I All Topics Except Wages*. 1941 Edition: Bulletin 694. Washington: United States Government Printing Office.

United States Department of Labor. 1948. *Workers Budgets in the United States: City Families and Single Persons, 1946 and 1947*. Bulletin No. 297. Washington: United States Department of Labor.

U.S. Department of Labour. 2006. 100 Years of U.S. *Consumer Spending: Data for the Nation, New York City and Boston*. Report 991.

Wells, Kathryn. 2013. "Annette Kellerman – the modern swimmer for modern women". Australian Government. http://www.australia.gov.au/about-australia/australian-story/annette-kellerman.

Woman's Institute of Domestic Arts and Sciences. 1925. *Designing and Planning Clothes: The Principles of Design Illustrated and Explained in Their Practical Application to Correct Dress for All Types*. Scranton: Bramcost Publications reproduced in facsimile 2008. ISBN: 9781934268704.

Woman's Institute of Domestic Arts and Sciences Ltd. *Harmony in Dress: the charm of beautiful clothes, good taste in dress, dress foundations, linen in figure and dress, color, its theory and application, fabrics and their adaptability, clothes suitability, good taste in millinery and accessories, planning wardrobes*. London.

Wright, Carroll. D. (ed.) 1903. *Bulletin of the Bureau of Labour: Volume VIII*. Department of Commerce and Labor. Washington: Government Printing Office.

Wright, Helen Russell. 1932. "A Year's Expenditures of Ten Railroad Laborers." *Social Service Review* 6 (1): 55-82.

Young, William. H. and Nancy K. Young. 2004. *The 1950s*. Westport: Greenwood Publishing Group.

Zimmerman, Carle C. 1935. "Laws of Consumption and Living" *American Journal of Sociology* 41 (1): 13-30.

Index

Accessories 95, 112, 131
    capsule wardrobe.....173
    cluster wardrobe......171
    colour 119
    outfit 133
    proportions...............116
    purchasing principles
       154
    research.....................217
    shopping....................119
    wardrobe review......167
Acetate...........................15
    care of.......................240
    characteristics 192
Acrylic 79
Adrian, Gilbert 59
Aeroplanes
    1900s..........................14
    1920s..........................38
    dress code 198
Age
    clothing 107
    hats............................227
Artificial Silk......*see* Rayon
Bags
    1920s..........................45
    1930s..........................58
    1940s..........................64
    1950s..........................86
    appropriateness.......103, 104
    caring for...................237
    outfit 133
    personality type 121
    storage 165
Balenciaga, Cristóbal......85

Banton, Travis.................59
Beauty 111, 251
    face............................ 248
    hands......................... 249
Black Tie Dress Codes 199
Blouses..................*see* Tops
Bocher, Main...................59
Body Proportions . 114, *see also* Greek proportions
Body Shape........... 112, 246
Budget .....*see also* Clothing Expenditure
    and 1928 prices 90
    hats............................ 225
    how much 90
    includes what.............91
    modern day example
        137
    splitting it 92
    value
        best for money.......94
        other kinds 96
Business Dress Codes . 200
Capsule Wardrobes
    capsule 172
    cluster 170
    minimalist 174
Capucci, Roberto............86
Cardigans.......see Sweaters
Care
    eye............................. 248
    face............................ 247
    feet............................ 249
    hair............................ 248
    hands......................... 249
    hats............................ 235

teeth............................248
Carnegie, Hattie 72
Carriage 247
Cars
   1900s 14
   1910s 26
   1920s 38
   1930s 50
   1940s 64
Cashin, Bonnie................85
Casual Dress Codes......200
Chanel, Gabrielle
   ("Coco")................46, 86
Clothing
   appropriateness
      age..........................107
      career 103
      climate 101
      faintheartedness ..108
      health 105
      leisure...................104
      modern day example
        138
      pregnancy.............105
      region 102
      willingness to care
         for.....................100
   care 237
      before you dress ..237
      colour....................241
      dry cleaning 241
      fabrics 239
      freezing.................243
      hand washing 242
      ironing...................242
      repairs 239
      spot cleaning 238
      when you get home
        237
   expenditure
      1900s.......................20
      1910s 30
      1920s.......................43
      1930s........................56
      1940s.......................69
      1950s.......................84
   purchasing
      criteria..................127
      records 150
Cocktail Dress...............201
Colour
   analogous scheme 118
   and lighting conditions
     118
   care of......................241
   characterisitcs 117
   colour wheel.............117
   complementary scheme
     118
   cool 117
   hair.............................119
   hats.............................227
   hue 117
   intensity 117
   monochromatic scheme
     118
   neutral scheme 118
   palette.......................119
   pastels.......................118
   personality 119
   retiring......................118
   schemes....................118
   shade.........................117
   the best 119
   tint.............................117
   value 117
   warm..........................117
Confidence
   developing 122
cost per wear 94
Cotton
   1910s............................26
   1920s............................39
   1930s................. 51, 52
   1940s............................65
   1950s............................80

appropriateness........101
care of......................240
characteristics 192
Cycles
   fashion......................131
   favourite...................130
   replacement..............130
Dacron 79
Daywear 7
   1900s..........................16
   1920s.................... 38, 45
   1930s..........................51
   1940s.................... 71, 72
   1950s..........................84
   and need........... 128, 129
   budget..........................95
Diet................................250
Dior, Christian 73
Disaster
   1900s..........................12
   1910s..........................24
   1920s..........................36
   1930s..........................48
   1950s..........................76
Doing the Laundry *see also* Clothing Care
   1900s..........................17
   1910s..........................28
   1920s..........................42
   1930s..........................55
   1940s..........................68
   1950s..........................82
Domestic Developments
   1900s..........................13
   1910s..........................24
   1920s..........................36
   1930s..........................49
   1940s..........................62
   1950s..........................77
Dralon 79
Dress Code
   aeroplane travel 198
   afternoon dress 198
   black tie 199
   business 200
   casual 200
   cocktail 201
   dinner party............. 201
   festive 202
   funerals..................... 202
   job interview 203
   lounge 203
   meeting the in-laws 203
   morning dress.......... 203
   Race Meetings 204
   religious services..... 205
   school........................ 205
   semi-formal.............. 205
   shows 206
   tea dress 206
   weddings 207
   white tie 207
Dresses
   fit 186
   outfit 132
   poorly made............. 195
   quality....................... 193
Dry Cleaning..241, *see also* Clothing Care
   after care 241
   repairs and alterations
      241
   stains......................... 241
Duff-Gordon, Lady Lucy
   ....*see* Lucile
Dynel................................65
Elastomer........................79
Electricity Supply
   1910s..........................29
   1920s..........................42
   1930s..........................55
   1940s..........................68
   1950s..........................82
Eveningwear .... 7, *see also* Good Clothes
   1920s..................... 38, 45

1940s 64, 72
1950s 85
and need....................128
and personality 122
capsule.......................174
care of........................100
cluster........................170
fabrics........................192
for a show 206
modern day example
....................................142
on a budget 95
purpose 132
spirit 132
theme.........................132
underwear.................133
Everyday Clothes.......... *see* Daywear
Exercise 251
Eye Care 248
Fabric Developments
1900s 15
1910s 26
1920s 39
1930s 52
1940s 65
1950s 79
Face
care 247
hats.............................228
Faintheartedness
and style....................122
Fath, Jacques 85
Fit 177
balanced waist..........179
breasts 178
dresses.......................186
freedom of movement
....................................181
general.......................180
Greek proportions...178
hats.............................234
hips 180

importance of 177
jackets........................183
learn more.................182
long waist..................179
pants 185
personality 178
shoes..........................186
short waist 179
signature waist 180
skirts 184
standard sizes .. 177, 181
sweaters 185
tops 185
underwear.................186
waist...........................179
Foot Care........................249
Formal Dress.*see* Black Tie
Fortuny, Mariano 33
Freezing..........................243
Funeral Dress................202
Fur
1920s...........................45
1930s...........................51
1940s...........................63
Gas Supply
1910s...........................29
1920s...........................42
1930s...........................55
1940s...........................68
1950s...........................82
Givenchy, Hubert de 86
Good Clothes 43, 129, 144, *see also* Eveningwear
Greek Proportions
interesting divisions 115
law of space division
....................................114
outfit divisions 115
Hair
1920s...........................45
1930s...........................51
1940s...........................64
1950s...........................78

and colour 118
and style 111
budgeting for 92
care 248
colour 119
hats 232
perming 1900s 14
perming 1930s 51
perming 1940s 64
perming 1950s 78
Hand Care 249
Hand Washing 242
Hats
   1900s 14
   1910s 26, 32
   1920 riots 108
   1920s 38, 45
   1930s 50, 58
   1940s 64, 72
   1950s 79
   age 227
   anatomy 224
   appropriateness 101, 102, 103, 104
   body 233
   brim 224
   budget 225
   care 235
   choosing 223
   colour 227
   crown 224
   face 228
   face shape 229
   fit 234
   hair 232
   handling 234
   outfit 133, 226
   purpose 225
   storing 234
   trim 224
Historical Clothing Styles 7
Hosiery
   outfit 133
Housing
   1900s 16
   1910s 27
   1920s 41
   1930s 54
   1940s 67
   1950s 81
How to Choose a Hat .. 223
Ideal Wardrobe
   1918 128
   1936 128
Income
   1900s 19
   1910s 30
   1920s 43
   1930s 55
   1940s 69
   1950s 83
Insect Repellent .. 164, 166, 238
Ironing 242
   1900s 18
   willingness to 101
Jackets
   fit 183
   poorly made 195
   proportions 184
   quality 193
Jersey
   1910s 25
   1920s 46
   1950s 86
Jewellery
   1910s 25
   1920s 40
   1950s 86
   appropriateness 103
   best value 95
   budget 92
   outfit 133
   style 113
Job Interview Dress 203
Klein, Anne 85

Lanvin, Jeanne 34
Laundry .... *see* Doing the Laundry
Linen
    1910s 26
    1920s 39
    1930s 51
    appropriateness 101
    care of 241
    characteristics 192
Lingerie ..... *See* underwear
Lounge Dress Code 203
Lucile 34
Madame Gres 72
Magazine Spread Technique 113, 119, 122, 163, 218
Makeup
    1920s 39
    1930s 51
    1940s 64
    1950s 79
    and fabric care 239
    and natural colouring 119
    and style 111
    budgeting for 92
    financial records 152
    for shopping 219
Manufacturing
    1900s 16
    1910s 26
    1920s 40
    1930s 53
    1940s 66
    1950s 80
McCardell, Clair 72
Meanwhile at Home
    1900s 16
    1910s 27
    1920s 41
    1930s 54
    1940s 67
    1950s 81
Mistakes 132, 162, 163
    understanding 150
Modacrylic 65
Mood Board .124, 125, 157
Mourning Dress 204
Nylon
    1930s 52
    1940s 65
Olefin 65
ON THE WORLD STAGE
    1900S 12
    1910s 24
    1920s 36
    1930s 48
    1940s 62
    1950s 76
Orlon 79
Other News
    1910 25
    1920s 37
    1930s 50
    1940s 63
Outfit
    "good" 104
    building 131
    confidence 122
    cost 90
    hats 226
    modern day example 134
    personality 134
    proportions 115
    signatures 123
    theme 132, 134
Pants
    1900s 21
    1920s 38, 46
    1940s 63, 64, 71
    1950s 85
    fit 185
    poorly made 195
    quality 193

storage 165
Paquin, Jeanne 21
Patou, Jean 46
Personal Brand .... see Signature
Personality
    colour 119
    fit 178
    purchasing principles
    122
    type 1 120
    type 2 120
    type 3 120
    type 4 120
    waist 180
Poiret, Paul 21, 46
Politics
    1900s 12
    1910s 24
    1920s 36
    1930s 48
    1950s 76
Polyester 65
    1950s 79, 85
Posture 246
Pregnancy 105
Professional Dress Code
    .... see Business
Pucci, Emilio 86
Purchasing Principles . 123, 124, 153
    and personality 122
Purse .... see Bags
Quality 189
    acetate 192
    and price 189
    appearance 192
    appropriateness 190
    budget 190
    comfort 193
    cotton 192
    durability 193
    fabrics 191
    flexibility 190
    form and function ... 189
    indicators of poor
        quality 195
    linen 192
    rayon 192
    silk 191
    style 190
    variability 190
    well made 190
    wool 192
Race Meeting Dress Code
    204
Rationing
    First World War 25
    hats 64
    Second World War 63
    UK end 70
    UK start 69
    US end 70
Rayon 15, 39
    1910s 26
    1930s 52
    1950s 80
    care of 240
    characteristics 192
Records
    clothing 150
    financial 152
    frequency of wear ... 151
    purchasing principles
    153
    replacement schedule
    151
Religious Service Dress
    Codes 205
Repairs 239, 241
Schiaparelli, Elsa 59
Schuberth, Emilio 85
Science and Technology
    1900s 12
    1910s 24
    1920s 36

1930s 49
1940s 62
1950s 77
Semi-Formal Dress Code
.... 205
Sewing Machines
   1900s 15
   1910s 26
   1920s 40
   1930s 52
   1940s 65
   1950s 80
Shoes
   1920s 39
   1930s 58
   1935 replacement cycle
      152
   1940s 64
   appropriateness 102, 104
   caring for 237, 243
   fit 186
   foot care 249
   freezing 243
   manufacturer consistency 187
   outfit 133
   quality 195
   repair 243
   shopping 219
   storage 166
Shopping 209
   designer collections. 212
   don't buy 219
   goals 209
   Greek proportions ... 213
   new clothes 215
   on the day 218
   principles 212
   research 217
   shoes 219
   sticking to the plan .. 210
   trying clothes on 220
   what can go wrong .. 210
   what to bring 219
   what to wear 218
   when to 213
   where to 214
Shopping List 154
   and replacement schedule 151
   buy what you will use
      134
   detail required 143
   ease of use 144
   flexibility 145
   leave space 145
   modern day example
      141
Silk
   1910s 26
   1920s 39
   1930s 51, 52
   1940s 65
   1950s 80
   appropriateness 101
   care of 240
   characteristics 191
Silk (artificial) ...*see* Rayon
Skirts
   fit 184
   poorly made 195
   proportions 184
   quality 193
SOCIAL AND TECHNOLOGICAL DEVELOPMENTS IN FASHION
   1900s 13
   1910s 25
   1920s 37
   1930s 50
   1940s 63
   1950s 78
Social Expectations
   1900s 13
   1910s 25
   1920s 37

1930s............................50
1940s............................63
1950s............................78
Sportswear
   1920s..........................38
   1930s..........................58
   1940s................... 65, 72
   care of.......................242
   Patou...........................46
Stockings
   1940s DIY 64
   nylon..................... 65, 84
   rayon...........................65
   silk......................... 39, 53
Streetwear............ 7, 84, 91
   and budget 95
   caring for..................237
Stress Management 252
Style
   body shape................112
   colour 116
   confidence 122
   foundation of............112
   keywords...................124
   learning 124
   levelling up 124
   modern day example
     140
   personality 120
   signature...................123
   what it is....................112
Summer Clothing
   appropriateness........102
   budgeting for 102
   colours.......................119
   provision for.............129
   purchasing principles
     153
   records 151
   value 96
   wardrobe review.......160
Sweaters
   fit 185

poorly made............. 195
quality...................... 193
Swimming
   for exercise 251
Swimwear
   1900s............................14
   1910s............................26
   1920s............................39
   1930s............................51
   1940s............................64
   1950s............................80
Teeth Care.................... 248
Telephone
   1920s............................43
   1930s............................55
   1940s............................69
   1950s............................83
Terylene 79
The Arts
   1900s............................13
   1910s............................25
   1920s............................37
   1930s............................49
   1940s............................62
   1950s............................77
Tops
   fit 185
   poorly made............. 195
   proportions.............. 185
   quality...................... 193
Trousers...............see Pants
Trousseau 206
Trying Clothes On....... 220
   cloth......................... 220
   colour....................... 220
   cut 221
Underwear
   1920s............................45
   cotton..........................84
   eveningwear 133
   fit 186
   outfit 133
   poorly made............. 195

quality 193
woollen 50, 84
Utility Scheme ... 66, 70, 71
Vionnet, Madeleine . 33, 59
Viscose .... *see* Rayon
Waist
   personality 180
War
   1900s 12
   1910s 24
   1920s 36
   1930s 48
   1940s 62
   1950s 76
Wardrobe Plan
   1935 advice 132
   basic needs 129
   duration 149
   problem 2
   purchasing principles
     153
   revisions 129
Wardrobe Review 159
   preparation 161
   when 160
   why 159
Water Supply
   1900s 17
   1910s 27
   1920s 41
   1930s 54
   1940s 68
   1950s 81
Weddings Dress Code . 207
White Tie Dress Code . 207
Winter 101
Winter Clothing
   appropriateness 103
   budgeting for 102

colours 119
provision for 129
purchasing principles
  153
records 151
wardrobe review 160
Womenswear
   Key Designers
     1900s 21
     1910s 33
     1920s 46
     1930s 59
     1940s 71
     1950s 85
   Key Figures
     1900s 21
     1910s 33
     1920s 46
     1930s 58
     1940s 71
     1950s 85
   Key Looks
     1900s 20
     1910s 32
     1920s 44
     1930s 57
     1940s 70
     1950s 84
Wool
   1910s 26
   1920s 39
   1930s 52
   1940s 71
   1950s 79
   appropriateness 101
   care of 240
   characteristics 192
   handwashing 242

Author's Note

Thanks again for buying my book.

If you'd like to let me know what you think, drop me a line at hello@alexandriablaelock.com.

Sifting through the historical detail from the first half of the twentieth century has been fascinating as well as enjoyable. There were tumultuous changes in style, fashion, and social expectations. When you add up all those changes, what we wear now suddenly makes a little more sense.

For some examples of appropriate and stylish outfits, visit alexandriablaelock.com/books/build-your-signature-wardrobe/ or my Pinterest board for other interesting information at pinterest.com.au/alexblaelock/build-your-signature-wardrobe/

For more, visit me at alexandriablaelock.com to:

- read my blog

- sign up for *Letters from my Library* to stay up to date on the development and release of my books. You'll also get research interestingness (that doesn't get to the blog), gossip about my writing life, and the odd special offer.

About the Author

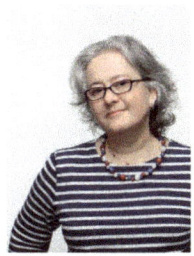

Alexandria Blaelock writes self-help books applying business techniques to personal matters like getting dressed, cleaning house, and feeding your friends.

She also writes short stories, some of them for *Ellery Queen's Mystery Magazine* and *Pulphouse Fiction Magazine*.

As a recovering Project Manager, she's probably too fond of sticking to plan. She lives in a forest because she enjoys birdsong, the scent of gum leaves and the sun on her face.

When not telecommuting to parallel universes from her Melbourne based imagination, she watches K-dramas, talks to animals, and drinks Campari. At the same time.

Discover more at www.alexandriablaelock.com.

www.ingramcontent.com/pod-product-compliance
Lightning Source LLC
Chambersburg PA
CBHW051543010526
44118CB00022B/2565